Alkaline Diet Cookbook for Two

2 Books in 1| Dr. Lewis's Meal Plan Project| Complete Guide on How to Eat Balanced Alkaline Foods for Him and Her (Premium Edition)

By Grace Lewis

Table of Contents

ALKALINE DIET COOKBOOK FOR WOMEN

Alkaline Diet Cookbook for Men

Alkaline Diet Cookbook for Women

Dr. Lewis's Meal Plan Project| How to Make Your Body Ready for Weight Loss by Balancing Acidic and Alkaline Foods

By Grace Lewis

Chapter 1 - Introduction

The alkaline diet is based on the consideration that a diet rich in acid foods ends up disturbing the acid-base balance of the body, promoting the loss of essential minerals, such as calcium and magnesium contained in the bones.

These alterations would favor the appearance of a chronic acidosis of mild degree, which in turn would be a predisposing factor for some diseases and for a general sense of malaise.

The alkaline diet recommends to consume 70-80% of alkaline foods and 20-30% of acid foods every day. This food model is much closer to the one followed by man until the discovery of agriculture than the current one.

The acidity of a food is not measured in its fresh state, but on the ashes (minerals) that remain after combustion. These inorganic substances, therefore not metabolizable, can behave as acids or bases, and as such participate in the maintenance of the normal organic pH.

Lemon, for example, has a very low pH, because of the abundant presence of citric acid; however, it is considered as an alkaline food because its acid components have an organic nature and as such they are easily metabolized by the body and eliminated with respiration, whereas the basic inorganic ones remain there for a longer time.

The elements that cause the formation of acids, by decreasing the urinary pH, are sulfur, phosphor and chlorine, whereas foods rich in sodium, potassium, magnesium and calcium are considered alkaline.

What do you eat on an alkaline diet?

The alkaline diet basically reinforces good, old-fashioned healthy eating. The diet recommends eating more vegetables, fruits and drinking plenty of water and cutting back on sugar, alcohol, meat and processed foods.

Where to start with the alkaline diet?

In this book you will find targeted recipes and especially easy to prepare to be able to approach the alkaline diet at its best.

At the end of the book you'll find my personal meal plan developed specifically for women, so that you can immediately experience the fantastic benefits that this diet can bring you.

Good luck and... Bon appetite!

Grace

Alkaline Diet Breakfast Recipes

1) Bowl of raspberry and banana smoothie

Preparation time:10 minutes   **Cooking time:** 10 minutes   **Servings: 2**

Ingredients:
- ✓ 2 cups fresh raspberries, split
- ✓ 2 large frozen bananas, peeled

Directions:
- ❖ In a blender, add the raspberries, bananas and almond milk and blend until smooth.

Nutrition: Calories

Ingredients:
- ✓ ½ cup of unsweetened almond milk
- ✓ 1/3 cup fresh mixed berries

- ❖ Transfer the smoothie to two serving bowls evenly.
- ❖ Top each bowl with berries and serve immediately.

2) Apple and walnut porridge

Preparation time: 10 minutes   **Cooking time:** 5 minutes   **Servings: 4**

Ingredients:
- ✓ 2 cups of unsweetened almond milk
- ✓ 3 tablespoons walnuts, chopped
- ✓ 3 tablespoons of sunflower seeds
- ✓ 2 large apples, peeled, pitted and grated

Directions:
- ❖ In a large skillet, stir together the milk, nuts, sunflower seeds, applesauce, vanilla and cinnamon over medium-low heat and cook for about 3-5 minutes, stirring often.

Nutrition: Calories

Ingredients:
- ✓ ½ teaspoon of organic vanilla extract
- ✓ Pinch of cinnamon powder
- ✓ ½ small apple, core and slices
- ✓ 1 small banana, peeled and sliced

- ❖ Remove from heat and transfer oatmeal to serving bowls.
- ❖ Top with apple and banana slices and serve.

3) Chia seed pudding

Preparation time: 10minutes   **Cooking time:** 10 minutes   **Servings: 3**

Ingredients:
- ✓ 2 cups of unsweetened almond milk
- ✓ ½ cup chia seeds
- ✓ 1 tablespoon maple syrup

Directions:
- ❖ In a large bowl, add the almond milk, chia seeds, maple syrup and vanilla extract and stir to combine well.

Nutrition: Calories

Ingredients:
- ✓ 1 teaspoon of organic vanilla extract
- ✓ 1/3 cup fresh strawberries, hulled and sliced
- ✓ 2 tablespoons of sliced almonds

- ❖ Cover the bowl and refrigerate for at least 3-4 hours, stirring occasionally.
- ❖ Serve with the strawberry and almond garnish.

4) Cauliflower and raspberry porridge

Preparation time: 10 minutes   **Cooking time:** 15 minutes   **Servings: 2**

Ingredients:
- ✓ 1 cup unsweetened coconut milk
- ✓ 1 cup cauliflower rice
- ✓ 1/3 cup fresh raspberries

Directions:
- ❖ In a skillet, add the coconut milk and cauliflower rice over medium heat and cook for about 2-3 minutes, stirring occasionally.

Nutrition: Calories

Ingredients:
- ✓ 3 tablespoons unsweetened coconut, shredded
- ✓ 3 drops of liquid stevia

- ❖ Add the raspberries and with the back of a spoon lightly crush them.
- ❖ Add the coconut and stevia and stir to combine.
- ❖ Cover the pan and cook for about 10 minutes, stirring occasionally.
- ❖ Serve hot.

5) Spicy quinoa porridge

Preparation time: 10 minutes   **Cooking time:** 15 minutes   **Servings: 4**

Ingredients:

- ✓ 1 cup uncooked, rinsed and drained red quinoa
- ✓ 2 cups of alkaline water
- ✓ ½ teaspoon of organic vanilla extract
- ✓ ½ cup of coconut milk

Directions:

- ❖ In a large skillet, mix the quinoa, water and vanilla extract over medium heat and bring to a boil.
- ❖ Reduce heat to low and simmer, covered for about 15 minutes or until all liquid is absorbed, stirring occasionally.

Nutrition: Calories

Ingredients:

- ✓ ¼ teaspoon fresh lemon peel, finely grated
- ✓ 10-12 drops of liquid stevia
- ✓ 1 teaspoon of cinnamon powder
- ✓ ½ teaspoon ground ginger
- ✓ Pinch of ground cloves
- ✓ 2 tablespoons of chopped almonds
- ❖ In the pan with the quinoa, add the coconut milk, lemon zest, stevia and spices and stir to combine.
- ❖ Immediately remove from heat and stir quinoa with a fork.
- ❖ Divide the quinoa mixture evenly among the serving bowls.
- ❖ Serve with a garnish of chopped almonds.

6) Chocolate quinoa porridge

Preparation time: 15 minutes   **Cooking time:** 30 minutes   **Servings: 4**

Ingredients:

- ✓ 1 cup uncooked quinoa, rinsed and drained
- ✓ 1 cup unsweetened almond milk
- ✓ 1 cup unsweetened coconut milk
- ✓ Pinch of sea salt

Directions:

- ❖ Heat a small nonstick skillet over medium heat and cook quinoa for about 3 minutes or until lightly toasted, stirring often.
- ❖ Add the almond milk, coconut milk and a pinch of salt and stir to combine.
- ❖ Increase heat to high and bring to a boil.

Nutrition: Calories

Ingredients:

- ✓ 2 spoons of cocoa powder
- ✓ 2 tablespoons of maple syrup
- ✓ ½ teaspoon of organic vanilla extract
- ✓ ½ cup fresh strawberries, hulled and sliced
- ❖ Reduce heat to low and cook, uncovered for about 20-25 minutes or until all liquid is absorbed, stirring occasionally.
- ❖ Remove from heat and immediately, stir in the cocoa powder, maple syrup and vanilla extract.
- ❖ Serve immediately with the garnish of strawberry slices.

7) Buckwheat porridge with walnuts

Preparation time: 15 minutes   **Cooking time:** 7 minutes   **Servings: 2**

Ingredients:

- ✓ ½ cup buckwheat
- ✓ 1 cup of alkaline water
- ✓ 2 tablespoons of chia seeds
- ✓ 15-20 almonds
- ✓ 1 cup unsweetened almond milk

Directions:

- ❖ In a large bowl, soak buckwheat groats in water overnight.
- ❖ In 2 other bowls, dip chia seeds and almonds, respectively.
- ❖ Drain the buckwheat and rinse well.
- ❖ In a nonstick skillet, add buckwheat and almond milk over medium heat and cook for about 7 minutes or until creamy.

Nutrition: Calories

Ingredients:

- ✓ ½ teaspoon of cinnamon powder
- ✓ 1 teaspoon of organic vanilla extract
- ✓ 3-4 drops of liquid stevia
- ✓ ¼ cup fresh mixed berries
- ❖ Drain chia seeds and almonds well.
- ❖ Remove the pan from the heat and stir in the almonds, chia seeds, cinnamon, vanilla extract and stevia.
- ❖ Serve warm with a berry garnish.

8) Fruity Oatmeal

Preparation time: 15 minutes   **Cooking time**: 10 minutes   Servings: 4

Ingredients:

- ✓ 4 cups of alkaline water
- ✓ 1 cup steel cut dry oats
- ✓ 1 large banana, peeled and mashed

Ingredients:

- ✓ 1½ cups of fresh mixed berries (your choice)
- ✓ ¼ cup walnuts, finely chopped

Directions:

- ❖ In a large skillet, add the water and oats over medium-high heat and bring to a boil.
- ❖ Reduce the heat to low and simmer for about 20 minutes, stirring occasionally.

Nutrition: Calories

- ❖ Remove from heat and cool slightly.
- ❖ Add the mashed banana and stir to combine.
- ❖ Top with strawberries and walnuts and serve.

9) Baked Walnut Oatmeal

Preparation time: 15 minutes   **Cooking time**: 45 minutes   Servings: 5

Ingredients:

- ✓ 1 tablespoon of flaxseed meal
- ✓ 3 tablespoons of alkaline water
- ✓ 3 cups of unsweetened almond milk
- ✓ ¼ cup maple syrup
- ✓ 2 tablespoons of coconut oil, melted and cooled
- ✓ 2 teaspoons of organic vanilla extract

Directions:

- ❖ Lightly grease an 8x8-inch baking dish. Set aside.
- ❖ In a large bowl, add the flaxseed meal and water and beat until well combined. Set aside for about 5 minutes.
- ❖ In the bowl of the flax mixture, add the remaining ingredients except the oats and nuts and mix until well combined.
- ❖ Add the oats and nuts and stir gently to combine.
- ❖ Place the mixture in the prepared baking dish and spread it out in an even layer.

Nutrition: Calories

Ingredients:

- ✓ 1 teaspoon of cinnamon powder
- ✓ 1 teaspoon of organic baking powder
- ✓ ¼ teaspoon of sea salt
- ✓ 2 cups of old rolled oats
- ✓ ½ cup almonds, chopped
- ✓ ½ cup walnuts, chopped

- ❖ Cover the pan with plastic wrap and refrigerate for about 8 hours.
- ❖ Preheat the oven to 350 degrees F. Arrange a rack in the center of the oven.
- ❖ Remove the pan from the refrigerator and let rest at room temperature for 15-20 minutes.
- ❖ Remove the plastic wrap and mix the oatmeal mixture well.
- ❖ Bake for about 45 minutes.
- ❖ Remove from oven and set aside to cool slightly.
- ❖ Serve hot.

10)   Banana Waffles

Preparation time: 15 minutes   **Cooking time**: 20 minutes   Servings: 5

Ingredients:

- ✓ 2 tablespoons of flax meal
- ✓ 6 tablespoons of warm alkaline water
- ✓ 2 bananas, peeled and mashed

Ingredients:

- ✓ 1 cup creamy almond butter
- ✓ ¼ cup whole coconut milk

Directions:

- ❖ In a small bowl, add the flax meal and warm water and whisk until well combined.
- ❖ Set aside for about 10 minutes or until mixture becomes thick.
- ❖ In a medium bowl, add bananas, almond butter and coconut milk, mix well.

Nutrition: Calories

- ❖ Add the flax meal mixture and stir until well combined.
- ❖ Preheat the waffle iron and grease it lightly.
- ❖ Place desired amount of batter in preheated waffle iron.
- ❖ Bake for about 3-4 minutes or until waffles turn golden brown.
- ❖ Repeat with the remaining mixture.
- ❖ Serve hot.

11)　Savory sweet potato waffles

Preparation time: 10 minutes　　　　**Cooking time**: 20 minutes　　　　**Servings: 2**

Ingredients:
- ✓ 1 medium sweet potato, peeled, grated and squeezed
- ✓ 1 teaspoon fresh thyme, chopped
- ✓ 1 teaspoon fresh rosemary, chopped

Ingredients:
- ✓ 1/8 teaspoon of red pepper flakes, crushed
- ✓ Sea salt and freshly ground black pepper, to taste

Directions:
- ❖ Preheat the waffle iron and then grease it.
- ❖ In a large bowl, add all ingredients and mix until well combined.

- ❖ Place ½ of the sweet potato mixture into the preheated waffle iron and bake for about 8-10 minutes or until golden brown.
- ❖ Repeat with the remaining mixture.
- ❖ Serve hot.

Nutrition: Calories

12)　Fruit Oatmeal Pancakes

Preparation time: 10 minutes　　　　**Cooking time**: 15 minutes　　　　**Servings: 3**

Ingredients:
- ✓ 1 cup rolled oats
- ✓ 1 medium banana, peeled and mashed
- ✓ ¼-½ cup unsweetened almond milk
- ✓ 1 tablespoon of organic baking powder

Ingredients:
- ✓ 1 tablespoon organic apple cider vinegar
- ✓ 1 tablespoon of agave nectar
- ✓ ½ teaspoon of organic vanilla extract
- ✓ ½ cup of fresh blackberries

- ❖ Immediately, cover the pan and cook for about 2-3 minutes or until golden brown.
- ❖ Flip the pancake and bake for another 1-2 minutes or until golden brown.
- ❖ Repeat with the remaining mixture.
- ❖ Serve hot.

Directions:
- ❖ Place all ingredients except blackberries in a large bowl and mix until well combined.
- ❖ Gently add the blackberries.
- ❖ Set the mixture aside for about 5-10 minutes.
- ❖ Preheat a large nonstick skillet over medium-low heat.
- ❖ Add about ¼ cup of the mixture and using a spatula, spread into an even layer.

Nutrition: Calories

13)　Tofu and mushroom muffins

Preparation time: 15 minutes　　　　**Cooking time**: 30 minutes　　　　**Servings: 6**

Ingredients:
- ✓ 1 teaspoon of olive oil
- ✓ 1½ cups fresh button mushrooms, chopped
- ✓ 1 shallot, chopped
- ✓ 1 teaspoon of minced garlic
- ✓ 1 teaspoon fresh rosemary, chopped
- ✓ Freshly ground black pepper, to taste

Directions:
- ❖ Preheat oven to 375 degrees F. Grease a 12-cup muffin pan.
- ❖ In a nonstick skillet, heat the oil over medium heat and sauté the shallots and garlic for about 1 minute.
- ❖ Add the mushrooms and cook for about 5-7 minutes, stirring often.
- ❖ Add the rosemary and black pepper and remove from heat.
- ❖ Set aside to cool slightly.
- ❖ In a food processor, add the tofu and remaining ingredients and pulse until smooth.

Ingredients:
- ✓ 1 (12.3ounce) package of firm silken tofu, drained, pressed and sliced
- ✓ ¼ cup unsweetened almond milk
- ✓ 2 tablespoons of nutritional yeast
- ✓ 1 tablespoon arrowroot starch
- ✓ ¼ teaspoon ground turmeric
- ✓ 1 teaspoon of coconut oil, softened
- ❖ Transfer the tofu mixture to a large bowl.
- ❖ Add the mushroom mixture.
- ❖ Divide the tofu mixture evenly among the prepared muffin cups.
- ❖ Bake for 20-22 minutes or until a toothpick inserted into the center comes out clean.
- ❖ Remove the muffin pan from the oven and place on a rack to cool for about 10 minutes.
- ❖ Carefully invert the muffins onto the wire rack and serve warm.

Nutrition: Calories

14)   Simple white bread

Preparation time: 10 minutes   **Cooking time**: 1 hour and 10 minutes   **Servings**: 8

Ingredients:
- ✓ 4 cups of spelt flour
- ✓ 4 tablespoons of sesame seeds
- ✓ 1 teaspoon of baking soda

Ingredients:
- ✓ ¼ teaspoon of sea salt
- ✓ 10-12 drops of liquid stevia
- ✓ 2 cups plus 2 tablespoons of unsweetened almond milk

Directions:
- ❖ Preheat oven to 350 degrees F. Line a 9x5-inch baking dish with greased baking paper.
- ❖ In a large bowl, add all ingredients and, using a fork, mix until well combined.
- ❖ Transfer the mixture to the prepared baking dish evenly.
- ❖ Bake for about 70 minutes or until a toothpick inserted into the center comes out clean.

- ❖ Remove from the oven and place the pan on a wire rack to cool for at least 10 minutes.
- ❖ Carefully flip the loaf onto the rack to cool completely before slicing.
- ❖ Using a sharp knife, cut the loaf into desired size slices and serve.

Nutrition: Calories

15)   Quinoa bread

Preparation time: 10 minutes   **Cooking time**: 1 hour and a half   **Servings**: 12

Ingredients:
- ✓ ¼ cup chia seeds
- ✓ 1 cup of alkaline water, divided by
- ✓ 1¾ cups uncooked quinoa, soaked overnight and rinsed
- ✓ ½ teaspoon of baking soda

Ingredients:
- ✓ ¼ teaspoon of sea salt
- ✓ ¼ cup olive oil
- ✓ 1 tablespoon fresh lemon juice

Directions:
- ❖ In a bowl, soak chia seeds in ½ cup of water overnight,
- ❖ Preheat oven to 320 degrees F. Line a baking sheet with baking paper.
- ❖ In a food processor, add the chia seed mixture and remaining ingredients and pulse for about 3 minutes.
- ❖ Place the bread mixture evenly in the prepared baking dish.
- ❖ Bake for about 1 1/2 hours or until a toothpick inserted into the center comes out clean.

- ❖ Remove the pan from the oven and place on a rack to cool for about 10 minutes.
- ❖ Carefully flip the loaf onto the rack to cool completely before slicing.
- ❖ Using a sharp knife, cut the loaf into desired size slices and serve.

Nutrition: Calories

16)   Zucchini and banana bread

Preparation time: 15 minutes   **Cooking time**: 45 minutes   **Servings**: 6

Ingredients:
- ✓ ½ cup almond flour, sifted
- ✓ 1½ teaspoons of baking soda
- ✓ ½ teaspoon of cinnamon powder
- ✓ ¼ teaspoon ground cardamom

Ingredients:
- ✓ 1/8 teaspoon of clove powder
- ✓ 1½ cups banana, peeled and sliced
- ✓ ¼ cup almond butter, softened
- ✓ 2 teaspoons of organic vanilla extract
- ✓ 1 cup zucchini, shredded and squeezed
- ❖ Gently add the grated zucchini.
- ❖ Pour the flour mixture evenly into the prepared baking dish.
- ❖ Bake for about 40-45 minutes or until a toothpick inserted into the center comes out clean.
- ❖ Remove from the oven and place the pan on a wire rack to cool for at least 10 minutes.
- ❖ Carefully flip the bread onto the rack to cool completely before slicing.

Directions:
- ❖ Preheat oven to 350 degrees F. Grease a 6x3-inch baking dish.
- ❖ In a large bowl, add the flour, baking soda and spices and with a fork, mix well.
- ❖ In another bowl, add the banana and use a fork to mash it completely.
- ❖ In the bowl of the banana, add the almond butter and vanilla extract and beat until well combined.
- ❖ Add the flour mixture and stir until just combined.

Nutrition: Calories

17) Granola with coconut, nuts and seeds

Preparation time: 15 minutes   **Cooking time**: 23 minutes   Servings: 8

Ingredients:

- ✓ ½ cup unsweetened coconut flakes
- ✓ 1 cup raw almonds
- ✓ 1 cup raw walnuts
- ✓ ½ cup raw, shelled sunflower seeds
- ✓ ¼ cup of coconut oil

Directions:

- ❖ Preheat oven to 275 F. Line a large baking sheet with baking paper.
- ❖ In a food processor, add the coconut flakes, almonds, nuts and seeds and pulse until finely chopped.
- ❖ Meanwhile, in a medium nonstick skillet, add the oil, maple syrup and vanilla extract and cook for 3 minutes over medium-high heat, stirring constantly.
- ❖ Remove from heat and immediately stir into the nut mixture.
- ❖ Transfer the mixture to the prepared baking sheet and spread evenly.
- ❖ Cook for about 25 minutes, stirring twice.

Nutrition: Calories

Ingredients:

- ✓ ½ cup maple syrup
- ✓ 1 teaspoon of organic vanilla extract
- ✓ ½ cup golden raisins
- ✓ ½ cup of black raisins
- ✓ Sea salt, to taste
- ❖ Remove the pan from the oven and immediately stir in the raisins.
- ❖ Sprinkle with a little salt.
- ❖ With the back of a spatula, flatten the surface of the mixture.
- ❖ Set aside to cool completely.
- ❖ Next, break the granola into uniform sized pieces.
- ❖ Serve this granola with your choice of non-dairy milk and fruit toppings.
- ❖ To store, transfer this granola to an airtight container and store in the refrigerator.

18) Tortilla Chips

Preparation time: **Cooking time**: 30 minutes   Servings: 8

Ingredients:

- ✓ 2 cups of Spelt Flour
- ✓ 1 teaspoon of Pure Sea Salt

Directions:

- ❖ Set the oven to 350 degrees Fahrenheit.
- ❖ Place spelt flour and pure salt in a food processor*. Blend for about 15 seconds.
- ❖ While stirring, slowly add the soybean oil until well combined.
- ❖ Continue to blend and slowly add Spring Water to a dough is formed.
- ❖ Prepare a work surface and cover it with a piece of parchment paper. Sprinkle the flour on it.
- ❖ Knead the dough for about 1 to 2 minutes, until just right.
- ❖ Cover a baking pan with a little Grape Seed Oil.

Nutrition: Calories

Ingredients:

- ✓ 1/2 cup of rinse water
- ✓ 1/3 cup of ground olive oil
- ❖ Place the prepared dart in the baking dish.
- ❖ Brush the mixture with a little grape oil and, if desired, a little pure sea salt.
- ❖ Cut dough into 8 pieces with a pizza knife.
- ❖ Bake for about 10-12 minutes or until the chips are starting toecome golden brown.
- ❖ Allow to cool before serving.
- ❖ Serve and enjoy your Tortilla Chips!

Helpful Hints: If you don't have a refrigerator, you can use a hand mixer or blender. However, you will get better results with an immersion blender. You can serve the Tortillas with our Sweet Barbecue Sauce, Guacamole, or "Cheese". Sauce .

19) Onion Rings

Preparation time: **Cooking time:** 30 Minutes.   **Servings:** 8

Ingredients:

- ✓ White onion or yellow onion
- ✓ 1 cup of Spelt Flour
- ✓ 1/2 cup of homemade Hempseed Milk
- ✓ 1/2 cup of Aquafaba *
- ✓ 2 teaspoons of Onion Powder.

Directions:

- ❖ Preheat our oven to 450 degrees Fahrenheit.
- ❖ Pour Homemade Hempseed Milk and Aquafaba into a medium bowl and mix well.
- ❖ Add 1 teaspoon of Oregano, 1 teaspoon of Onion Powder, 1/2 teaspoon of Cayenne, and 1 teaspoon of Pure Sea Salt to the wet ingredients and mix.
- ❖ Peel the Onions, slice the ends.
- ❖ Cut peeled onion into slices about 1/4 inch thick. Cut the onion into rings.
- ❖ Add the Spelt flour, 1 teaspoon of Oregano, 1 teaspoon of Onion Powder, 1/2 teaspoon of Cayenne, and 1
- ❖ taspoon of Pure Sea Salt in a container with a quart. Shake out all the liquid.

Nutrition: Calories

Ingredients:

- ✓ 2 teaspoons of Oregano
- ✓ 1 teaspoon of Cayenne powder
- ✓ 2 teaspoons of Pure Sea Salt
- ✓ 3 tablespoons of grape oil

- ❖ Brush a baking sheet with Grape Seed Oil 8. Place a couple onion rings over the water mixture.
- ❖ Put the water onion rings in the dry mixture and turn until coated on both sides.
- ❖ Place the covered onion rings on the baking sheet.
- ❖ Repeat steps 8 to 10 until all onion rings are covere.
- ❖ Lightly spray the rings with Grape seed oil.
- ❖ Water for about 10-15 minutes until it shines.
- ❖ This is all possible for coool them before serving.
- ❖ Serve and enjoy our onion rings!

Helpful Hints: If you haven't made Aquafaba, add 1/2 extra millet of Homemade hemp seed milk. You can use Onion rings with our sweet Bärbecue Sauce , or "Cheese" Sauce .

20) Strawberry Sorbet

Preparation time: 4 hours   **Cooking time:**   **Servings:** 4

Ingredients:

- ✓ 2 cups of Strawberries*.
- ✓ 1 1/2 teaspoons of spelt flour

Directions:

- ❖ Add the sugar Date, water and flour Spelt in a saucepan and simmer for about ten minutes. The mixture should look like a syrup.
- ❖ Remove the meat from the cap and let it rest.
- ❖ After cooling, add Strawberry puree and stir.
- ❖ Place this mixture in a container and freeze.

Nutrition: Calories

Ingredients:

- ✓ 1/2 cup of sugar Date
- ✓ 2 cups of Spring Water

- ❖ Cut it into pieces, put the butter in a bowl and beat until it reaches the limit.
- ❖ Place all the butter in the container and let it chill for at least four hours.
- ❖ Serve and enjoyy your Strawberry Sorbet!

Helpful hints: If you don't have fresh berries, you can use frozen ones.

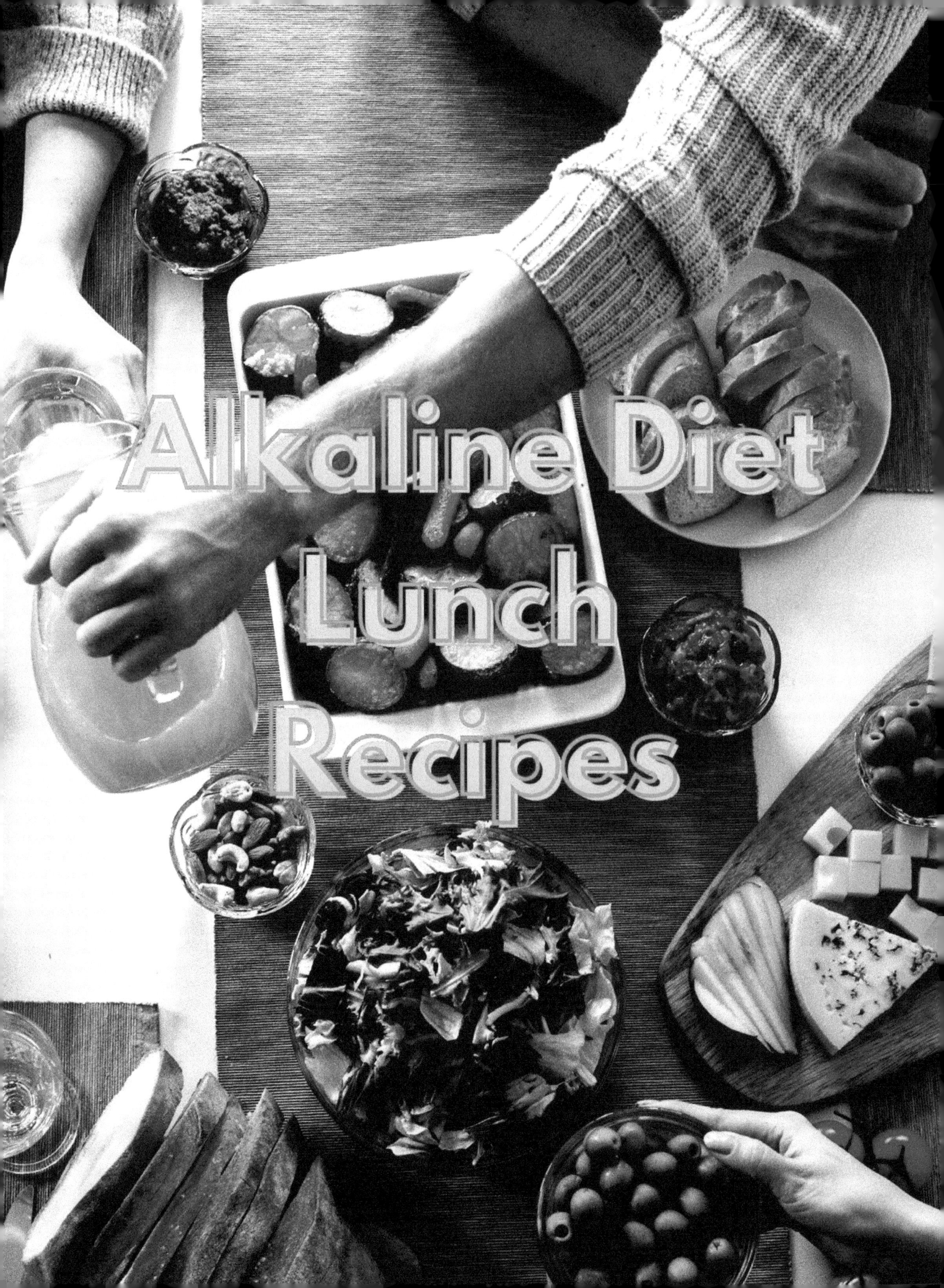

Alkaline Diet Lunch Recipes

21) Tomato and vegetable salad

Preparation time: 15 minutes.   **Cooking time**:   **Servings: 4**

Ingredients:
- ✓ 6 cups of fresh vegetables
- ✓ 2 cups of cherry tomatoes
- ✓ 2 shallots, chopped

Directions:
- ❖ Place all ingredients in a large bowl and mix to coat well.

Ingredients:
- ✓ 2 tablespoons of extra virgin olive oil
- ✓ 2 tablespoons fresh orange juice
- ✓ 1 tablespoon fresh lemon juice
- ❖ Cover the bowl and refrigerate for about 6-8 hours.
- ❖ Remove from refrigerator and mix well before serving.

Nutrition: Calories

22) Cauliflower Soup

Preparation time: 15 minutes   **Cooking time**: 30 minutes.   **Servings: 4**

Ingredients:
- ✓ 2 tablespoons of olive oil
- ✓ 1 yellow onion, chopped
- ✓ 2 carrots, peeled and cut into pieces
- ✓ 2 garlic cloves, minced
- ✓ 1 Serrano bell pepper, finely chopped
- ✓ 2 stalks of celery, chopped
- ✓ 1 teaspoon ground turmeric
- ✓ 1 teaspoon of ground coriander

Directions:
- ❖ Heat the oil over medium heat in a large soup pot and sauté the onion, carrot and celery for about 4-6 minutes.
- ❖ Add the garlic, serrano pepper and spices and sauté for about 1 minute.
- ❖ Add the cauliflower and cook for about 5 minutes, stirring occasionally.

Ingredients:
- ✓ 1 teaspoon of ground cumin
- ✓ ¼ teaspoon of red pepper flakes, crushed
- ✓ 1 head of cauliflower, chopped
- ✓ 4 cups of homemade vegetable broth
- ✓ 1 cup unsweetened coconut milk
- ✓ Sea salt and freshly ground black pepper, to taste
- ✓ 2 tablespoons fresh chives, finely chopped

- ❖ Add the broth and coconut milk and bring to a boil over medium-high heat.
- ❖ Reduce the heat to low and simmer for about 15 minutes.
- ❖ Season the soup with salt and black pepper and remove from heat.
- ❖ Using an immersion blender, blend the soup until smooth.
- ❖ Serve warm and garnish with chives.

Nutrition: Calories

23)   Tomato Soup

Preparation time: 15 minutes   **Cooking time**: 45 minutes   **Servings: 4**

Ingredients:
- ✓   2 tablespoons of coconut oil
- ✓   2 carrots, coarsely chopped
- ✓   1 large white onion, coarsely chopped
- ✓   3 garlic cloves, minced
- ✓   5 large tomatoes, coarsely chopped

Directions:
- ❖   Melt the coconut oil in a large soup pot over medium heat and cook the carrot and onion for about 10 minutes, stirring often.
- ❖   Add the garlic and sauté for about 1-2 minutes.
- ❖   Add the tomatoes, tomato paste, basil, broth, salt and black pepper and bring to a boil.

Nutrition: Calories

Ingredients:
- ✓   1 tablespoon of homemade tomato paste
- ✓   3 cups of homemade vegetable broth
- ✓   ¼ cup fresh basil, chopped
- ✓   ¼ cup unsweetened coconut milk
- ✓   Sea salt and freshly ground black pepper, to taste
- ❖   Reduce the heat to low and simmer uncovered for about 30 minutes.
- ❖   Add the coconut milk and remove from heat.
- ❖   Using an immersion blender, blend the soup until smooth.
- ❖   Serve hot.

24)   Garlic broccoli

Preparation time: 10 minutes   **Cooking time**: 8 minutes   **Servings: 2**

Ingredients:
- ✓   1 tablespoon of extra virgin olive oil
- ✓   3-4 garlic cloves, minced

Directions:
- ❖   Heat the oil over medium heat in a large skillet and sauté the garlic for about 1 minute.
- ❖   Add the broccoli and sauté for about 2 minutes.

Nutrition: Calories

Ingredients:
- ✓   2 cups of broccoli florets
- ✓   2 tablespoons of tamari
- ❖   Add the tamari and sauté for about 4-5 minutes or until desired doneness.
- ❖   Remove from heat and serve hot.

25)   Curried okra

Preparation time: 10 minutes   **Cooking time**: 15 minutes   **Servings: 3**

Ingredients:
- ✓   1 tablespoon of olive oil
- ✓   ½ teaspoon of cumin seeds
- ✓   ¾ lb okra pods, trimmed and cut into 2-inch pieces
- ✓   ½ teaspoon of curry powder

Directions:
- ❖   Heat oil in a large skillet over medium heat
- ❖   For about 30 seconds, sauté the cumin seeds
- ❖   Add the okra and sauté for about 1-1½ minutes.
- ❖   Reduce heat to low and cook covered for about 6-8 minutes, stirring occasionally.

Nutrition: Calories

Ingredients:
- ✓   ½ teaspoon of chili powder
- ✓   1 teaspoon of ground coriander
- ✓   Sea salt and freshly ground black pepper, to taste

- ❖   Add the curry powder, red pepper and cilantro and stir to combine.
- ❖   Increase the heat to medium and cook uncovered for another 2-3 minutes or so.
- ❖   Season with the salt and pepper and remove from heat.
- ❖   Serve hot.

26)   Mushrooms curry

Preparation time: 20 minutes   **Cooking time**: 20 minutes   **Servings: 4**

Ingredients:
- ✓ 2 cups of tomatoes, chopped
- ✓ 1 green chili pepper, chopped
- ✓ 1 teaspoon fresh ginger, chopped
- ✓ 2 tablespoons of olive oil
- ✓ ½ teaspoon of cumin seeds
- ✓ ¼ teaspoon ground coriander
- ✓ ¼ teaspoon ground turmeric

Directions:
- ❖ In a food processor, add the tomatoes, green chiles and ginger and pulse until it forms a smooth paste.
- ❖ Heat the oil in a skillet over medium heat.
- ❖ For about 1 minute, sauté the cumin seeds.
- ❖ Add the spices and sauté for about 1 minute.

Ingredients:
- ✓ ¼ teaspoon of chili powder
- ✓ 2 cups fresh shiitake mushrooms, sliced
- ✓ 2 cups fresh button mushrooms, sliced
- ✓ 1¼ cup of water
- ✓ ¼ cup unsweetened coconut milk
- ✓ Sea salt and freshly ground black pepper, to taste

- ❖ Add the tomato mixture and cook for about 5 minutes.
- ❖ Add the mushrooms, water and coconut milk and bring to a boil.
- ❖ Cook for about 10-12 minutes, stirring occasionally.
- ❖ Season with the salt and black pepper and remove from heat.
- ❖ Serve hot.

Nutrition: Calories

27)   Glazed Brussels sprouts

Preparation time: 15 minutes   **Cooking time**: 15 minutes   **Servings: 3**

Ingredients:
- ✓ 3 cups Brussels sprouts, cut and halved
- ✓ Sea salt, to taste
- ✓ 2 tablespoons of coconut oil, melted
- ✓ For the orange glaze:
- ✓ 1 tablespoon of coconut oil
- ✓ 2 small shallots, thinly sliced

Directions:
- ❖ Preheat oven to 400 degrees F. Line a baking sheet with baking paper.
- ❖ In a bowl, add the Brussels sprouts, a little salt and oil and toss to coat well.
- ❖ Transfer the mixture to the prepared baking dish.
- ❖ Roast for about 10-15 minutes, turning once halfway through.
- ❖ Meanwhile, prepare the frosting.
- ❖ In a skillet, melt the coconut oil over medium heat and sauté the scallions for about 5 minutes.
- ❖ Add the orange zest and sauté for about 1 minute.

Ingredients:
- ✓ 2 tablespoons of fresh orange zest, finely grated
- ✓ ¼ teaspoon ground ginger
- ✓ 2/3 cup fresh orange juice
- ✓ 1 tablespoon of sambal oelek (raw chili paste)
- ✓ 2 tablespoons of coconut amino acids
- ✓ 1 teaspoon of tapioca starch
- ✓ Sea salt, to taste
- ❖ Stir in the ginger, orange juice, sambal oelek and coconut amino acid and cook for about 5 minutes.
- ❖ Slowly add the tapioca starch, whisking constantly.
- ❖ Cook for about 2-3 minutes longer, stirring often.
- ❖ Add salt and remove from heat.
- ❖ Transfer roasted Brussels sprouts to a serving platter. Top evenly with the orange glaze.
- ❖ Serve immediately garnished with scallions.

Nutrition: Calories

28)   Sauteed mushrooms

Preparation time: 15 minutes   **Cooking time**: 16 minutes   **Servings: 2**

Ingredients:
- ✓ 2 tablespoons of olive oil
- ✓ ½ teaspoon cumin seeds, lightly crushed
- ✓ 2 medium onions, thinly sliced

Directions:
- ❖ Heat oil in a frying pan over medium heat
- ❖ For about 1 minute, sauté the cumin seeds.
- ❖ Add the onion and sauté for about 4-5 minutes.

Ingredients:
- ✓ ¾ lb fresh mushrooms, chopped
- ✓ Sea salt and freshly ground black pepper, to taste

- ❖ Add the mushrooms and sauté for about 5-7 minutes.
- ❖ Add the salt and black pepper and sauté for about 2-3 minutes.
- ❖ Remove from heat and serve hot.

Nutrition: Calories

29)   Sweet and sour cabbage

Preparation time: 10 minutes   **Cooking time**: 20 minutes   **Servings**: 4

Ingredients:
- ✓ 1 tablespoon of extra virgin olive oil
- ✓ 1 lemon, with seeds and thinly sliced
- ✓ 1 onion, chopped
- ✓ 3 garlic cloves, minced

Directions:
- ❖ In a large skillet, heat the oil over medium heat and cook the lemon slices for about 5 minutes.
- ❖ Using a slotted spoon, remove the lemon slices.

Ingredients:
- ✓ 2 pounds of fresh cabbage, hard ribs removed and trimmed
- ✓ ½ cup shallots, chopped
- ✓ 1 tablespoon of agave nectar
- ✓ Sea salt and freshly ground black pepper, to taste
- ❖ In the same skillet, add the onion and garlic and sauté for about 5 minutes.
- ❖ Add the cabbage, scallions, agave nectar, salt and black pepper and cook for about 8-10 minutes, stirring occasionally.
- ❖ Remove from heat and serve hot.

Nutrition: Calories

30)   Brussels sprouts with walnuts

Preparation time: 15 minutes   **Cooking time**: 15 minutes   **Servings**: 2

Ingredients:
- ✓ ½ pound Brussels sprouts, halved
- ✓ 1 tablespoon of olive oil
- ✓ 2 garlic cloves, minced
- ✓ ½ teaspoon of red pepper flakes, crushed

Directions:
- ❖ Place a steamer basket in a large pot of boiling water.
- ❖ Place Brussels sprouts in the basket of the steamer and steam, covered for about 6-8 minutes.
- ❖ Drain Brussels sprouts well.
- ❖ In a large skillet, heat the oil over medium heat and sauté the garlic and red pepper flakes for about 40 seconds.

Ingredients:
- ✓ Sea salt and freshly ground black pepper, to taste
- ✓ 1 tablespoon fresh lemon juice
- ✓ 1 tablespoon pine nuts

- ❖ Add the Brussels sprouts, salt and black pepper and sauté for about 4-5 minutes.
- ❖ Add the lemon juice and sauté for about 1 minute more.
- ❖ Add pine nuts and remove from heat.
- ❖ Serve hot.

Nutrition: Calories

31)   Roasted Butternut Squash

Preparation time: 15 minutes   **Cooking time**: 45 minutes   **Servings**: 6

Ingredients:
- ✓ 8 cups butternut squash, peeled, seeded and diced
- ✓ 2 tablespoons of melted almond butter
- ✓ ½ teaspoon ground cinnamon

Directions:
- ❖ Preheat oven to 425 degrees F. Place foil pieces on 2 baking sheets.
- ❖ In a large bowl, add all ingredients and mix to coat well.

Ingredients:
- ✓ ½ teaspoon of ground cumin
- ✓ ¼ teaspoon of red pepper flakes
- ✓ Sea salt, to taste
- ❖ Arrange the pumpkin pieces on the prepared baking sheets in a single layer.
- ❖ Roast for about 40-45 minutes.
- ❖ Remove from oven and serve.

Nutrition: Calories

32)   Broccoli with peppers

Preparation time: 15 minutes   **Cooking time**: 10 minutes   **Servings**: 4

Ingredients:
- ✓ 2 tablespoons of olive oil
- ✓ 4 garlic cloves, minced
- ✓ 1 large white onion, sliced
- ✓ 2 cups of small broccoli florets

Directions:
- ❖ In a large skillet, heat the oil over medium heat and sauté the garlic for about 1 minute.

Ingredients:
- ✓ 3 red peppers, seeded and sliced
- ✓ ¼ cup homemade vegetable broth
- ✓ Sea salt and freshly ground black pepper, to taste

- ❖ Add the onion, broccoli and peppers and sauté for about 5 minutes.
- ❖ Add the broth and sauté for about 4 more minutes.
- ❖ Serve hot.

33)   Shrimp with tamari

Preparation time: 15 minutes   **Cooking time**: 6 minutes   **Servings**: 2

Ingredients:
- ✓ 1 tablespoon of olive oil
- ✓ 2 garlic cloves, minced
- ✓ ½ pound of raw, peeled and deveined jumbo shrimps

Directions:
- ❖ In a large skillet, heat the oil over medium heat and sauté the garlic for about 1 minute.

Nutrition: Calories

Ingredients:
- ✓ 2 tablespoons of tamari
- ✓ Freshly ground black pepper, to taste

- ❖ Stir in the shrimp, tamari and black pepper and cook for about 4-5 minutes or until completely done.
- ❖ Serve hot.

34)   Vegetarian Kebab

Preparation time: 20 minutes   **Cooking time**: 10 minutes   **Servings**: 4

Ingredients:
  For the marinade:
- ✓ 2 garlic cloves, minced
- ✓ 2 teaspoons fresh basil, chopped
- ✓ 2 teaspoons fresh oregano, chopped
- ✓ ½ teaspoon of cayenne pepper
- ✓ Sea salt and freshly ground black pepper, to taste
- ✓ 2 tablespoons fresh lemon juice

Directions:
- ❖ For the marinade: in a large bowl, add all ingredients and mix until well combined.
- ❖ Add the vegetables to the marinade and toss to coat well.
- ❖ Cover and refrigerate to marinate the vegetables for at least 6-8 hours.
- ❖ In a large bowl of water, soak the wooden skewers for at least 30 minutes.

Nutrition: Calories

Ingredients:
- ✓ 2 tablespoons of olive oil
  For vegetables:
- ✓ 2 large zucchini, cut into thick slices
- ✓ 8 large button mushrooms, quartered
- ✓ 1 yellow bell pepper, seeded and diced
- ✓ 1 red bell pepper, seeded and diced

- ❖ Preheat grill to medium-high heat. Generously grease the grill grate.
- ❖ Remove the vegetables from the bowl and discard the marinade.
- ❖ Thread the vegetables onto the pre-soaked wooden skewers, starting with the zucchini, mushrooms and peppers.
- ❖ Grill for about 8-10 minutes or until cooked through, turning occasionally.

35)   Fried onion sprout

Preparation time: 5 minutes   **Cooking time**: 10 minutes   **Servings**: 4

Ingredients:
- ✓ 2½ pounds Brussels sprouts, cut 4 slices bacon, cut into 1-inch pieces
- ✓ 1 tablespoon of extra virgin coconut oil
- ✓ 1 tomato, chopped
- ✓ 1 onion, chopped

Directions:
- ❖ Add sprouts to boiling water in a pot.
- ❖ Let them cook for about 3-5 minutes.
- ❖ Drain and set aside.
- ❖ Saute onions in a greased skillet for 4 minutes.

Nutrition: Calories

Ingredients:
- ✓ 4 sprigs of thyme or savory, divided
- ✓ 1 teaspoon celtic sea salt, iodine-free
- ✓ Freshly ground pepper to taste
- ✓ 2 teaspoons of lemon juice (optional)

- ❖ Mix with salt, pepper and thyme
- ❖ Add the drained sprouts to the skillet and stir for 3 minutes.
- ❖ Remove and discard sprigs of grasses.
- ❖ Serve warm with lemon juice and chopped spring onion on top.

36)   Southwestern stuffed sweet potatoes

Preparation time: **Cooking time:**   **Portions:**

Ingredients:

- ✓ Sliced avocado (1)
- ✓ Pinch of cumin
- ✓ Pinch of dried red chili flakes
- ✓ Spinach (3 c.)
- ✓ Sliced shallot (1)
- ✓ Black beans (.5 c.)
- ✓ Coconut oil (2 tablespoons)
- ✓ Sweet potatoes

Directions:

- ❖ Turn on the oven and give it time to heat up to 400 degrees. Clean the sweet potatoes and pierce them a few times with a fork.
- ❖ Add baking paper to a baking sheet and place sweet potatoes on top. Add to the oven to bake.
- ❖ After 50 minutes, the potatoes should be soft. Remove them from the oven and give them time to cool.
- ❖ Meanwhile, take a skillet and add the coconut oil along with the black beans and shallots.

Nutrition: Calories

Ingredients:

- ✓ Drugs
- ✓ Pepper and salt
- ✓ Chopped coriander (1 handful)
- ✓ Cumin (1 teaspoon)
- ✓ Lime Juice (1)
- ✓ Olive oil (3 tablespoons)

- ❖ Cook these for a few minutes before adding the cumin, chili flakes and spinach, stirring to mix well.
- ❖ Finally, take a small bowl and whisk the ingredients for the dressing well.
- ❖ Cut the sweet potatoes in half before stuffing them with the black bean mixture you made.
- ❖ Add a few slices of avocado and some of the dressing poured over before serving.

37)   Zoodles with cream sauce

Preparation time: **Cooking time:**   **Portions:**

Ingredients:

- ✓ Toasted pepitas (2 tablespoons)
- ✓ Pepper (.5 tsp.)
- ✓ Salt (1 teaspoon)
- ✓ Chopped coriander (2 tablespoons)
- ✓ Water (1 tablespoon)

Directions:

- ❖ Add a little coconut oil to melt in a skillet before adding the zucchini noodles. Cook for 5 minutes before turning off the heat.
- ❖ Take out a blender and combine together the pepper, salt, 1 tablespoon cilantro, water, lemon juice, oil and avocado. Mix well and cook to make the cream.

Nutrition: Calories

Ingredients:

- ✓ Lemon juice (.5)
- ✓ Olive oil (2 tablespoons)
- ✓ Pitted avocado (1)
- ✓ Spiral zucchini (1)
- ✓ Coconut oil (1 tablespoon)
- ❖ Add the sauce to the skillet with the noodles and stir to combine. Move to a serving bowl and add the rest of the cilantro and toasted pepitas before serving.

38)   Rainbow Pad Thai

Preparation time: **Cooking time:**   **Portions:**

Ingredients:

- ✓ Avocado cubes (1)
- ✓ Chopped coriander (1 c.)
- ✓ Shredded daikon radish (1 c.)
- ✓ Chopped broccoli (1 c.)
- ✓ Shredded red cabbage (1 c.)
- ✓ Sliced shallots (3)
- ✓ Shredded carrots (2)
- ✓ Spiral Zucchini (3)

Directions:

- ❖ Add ingredients for Pad Thai, except avocado, to a large bowl and mix.
- ❖ Blend together all the ingredients you have for the dressing until creamy and combined.

Nutrition: Calories

Ingredients:

- For the dressing
- ✓ Chopped ginger (1 teaspoon)
- ✓ Chopped garlic clove (1)
- ✓ Sesame oil (1 tablespoon)
- ✓ Tahini (.25 c.)
- ✓ Lime Juice (1)

- ❖ Top the vegetables with the diced avocado and pour the dressing over them before serving.

39) Lentils and vegetables

Preparation time: **Cooking time:**   **Portions:**

Ingredients:
- ✓ Avocado (1)
- ✓ Crushed almonds (1 tablespoon)
- ✓ Crushed black pepper (1 teaspoon)
- ✓ Salt (1 teaspoon)
- ✓ Arugula (1 c.)
- ✓ Brown or green lentils (.5 c.)

Directions:
- ❖ Add the vegetable broth to a skillet over medium heat. Let it begin to simmer before adding the lemon juice, carrot, broccoli and pak choi.

Nutrition: Calories

Ingredients:
- ✓ Cooked wild rice (1 c.)
- ✓ Lemon juice (.5)
- ✓ Diced Carrot (1)
- ✓ Broccoli florets (.5 c.)
- ✓ Sliced Pak choi (.5 c.)
- ✓ Vegetable stock (.25 c.)
- ❖ After 5 minutes, turn off the heat and stir in the almonds, pepper, salt, arugula, lentils and wild rice.
- ❖ Move this mixture to plates and top with a few slices of avocado before serving.

40) Vegetable dish with sesame

Preparation time: **Cooking time:**   **Portions:**

Ingredients:
- ✓ Sesame seeds (1 teaspoon)
- ✓ Lemon juice (.5)
- ✓ Tamari Sauce (2 tablespoons)
- ✓ Chopped garlic clove (1)
- ✓ Diced red bell pepper (.5 c.)

Directions:
- ❖ Heat half a tablespoon of sesame oil and one tablespoon of olive oil in a skillet. Add the tofu and let it cook for a bit.
- ❖ After ten minutes, remove the tofu and add a little more of the two oils.

Nutrition: Calories

Ingredients:
- ✓ Finely chopped broccoli florets (2 c.)
- ✓ Cubed tofu (8 ounces)
- ✓ Olive oil (2 tablespoons)
- ✓ Sesame oil, toasted (1.5 tablespoons)

- ❖ Stir in the garlic, red bell bell pepper and broccoli until they soften a bit. Add the tofu and stir in the lemon juice and soy sauce as well.
- ❖ Top this dish with a few sesame seeds before serving.

Alkaline Diet Dinner Recipes

41)   Stew without beef

Preparation time: Cooking time: Servings: 4

Ingredients:
- ✓ Dried oregano, 1 teaspoon
- ✓ Celery, diced, 2 stalks
- ✓ Large diced potato
- ✓ Sliced carrot, 3 c.
- ✓ Water, 2 c.
- ✓ Vegetable broth, 3 c.

Directions:
- ❖ Heat the avocado oil in a top pan. Put in the pepper, salt, garlic cloves and onion bulbs. Cook everything for two to three minutes, or until the onion is soft.
- ❖ Add the bay leaf, oregano, celery, potato, carrot, water and broth. Allow to simmer, then lower the heat and prepare for 30-45 minutes, or until the carrots and potatoes become soft.

Nutrition: Calories

Ingredients:
- ✓ Pepper, one teaspoon
- ✓ Sea salt, one teaspoon
- ✓ Garlic puree, 2 bulbs
- ✓ Diced onion, 1 c.
- ✓ Avocado oil, 1 tablespoon
- ✓ Laurel
- ❖ Taste and adjust seasonings as needed. If it's too thick, you can add more water or broth.
- ❖ Divide among four bowls and enjoy.

42)   Emmenthal soup

Preparation time: Cooking time: Servings: 2

Ingredients:
- ✓ Cayenne
- ✓ Nutmeg
- ✓ Pumpkin seeds, 1 tablespoon
- ✓ Chopped chives, 2 tablespoons

Directions:
- ❖ Place the potato and cauliflower in a saucepan with the vegetable broth until tender.
- ❖ Place in a blender and blend.

Nutrition: Calories

Ingredients:
- ✓ Diced Emmenthal cheese, 3 tablespoons
- ✓ Vegetable broth, 2 c.
- ✓ Diced potato, 1
- ✓ Shredded cauliflower, 2 c.
- ❖ Add the spices and adjust to taste.
- ❖ Pour into bowls, add chives and cheese and mix well.
- ❖ Garnish with pumpkin seeds. Enjoy.

43)   Spaghetti with broccoli

Preparation time: Cooking time: Servings: 2

Ingredients:
- ✓ Pepper
- ✓ Halls
- ✓ Vegetable broth, 1 teaspoon
- ✓ Oregano plant, 1 teaspoon
- ✓ Lemon juice, 1 tablespoon
- ✓ Sliced carrots, 3
- ✓ Diced tomatoes, 3

Directions:
- ❖ Place a pot of water halfway up and add the salt. Allow to boil and add the pasta. Prepare according to box instructions. Empty.
- ❖ Place broccoli in another bowl and cover with h2O. Prepare for five minutes.
- ❖ Place a skillet over normal heat and put two tablespoons of olive oil in the pan and heat. Place the bulbs, garlic and onion in and prepare until soft and fragrant. Remove from the skillet and set aside.

Nutrition: Calories

Ingredients:
- ✓ Broccoli cut into florets, 1 head
- ✓ Sliced red bell pepper - bell, one
- ✓ Sliced onion bulb, one
- ✓ Diced garlic bulbs, two cloves
- ✓ EVOO, 4 tablespoons
- ✓ Buckwheat pasta, 1 lb.

- ❖ carrots. Cook for five minutes, then put in the sweet bell pepper and prepare for another five minutes, now put in the tomatoes and prepare for two minutes.
- ❖ Drain the broccoli completely and add it to the skillet with the rest of the vegetables. Return the onions and garlic to the skillet.
- ❖ Add the vegetable broth, oregano and lemon juice. Add a little pepper and salt, taste and adjust seasonings if needed. Stir well to combine.
- ❖ Place the cooked pasta on a serving plate. Pour over the vegetable mixture and toss to combine.

44)   Indian Lentil Curry

Preparation time: **Cooking time:**   Servings: 4 - 6

Ingredients:
- ✓ Lime Juice
- ✓ Chopped coriander
- ✓ Halls
- ✓ EVOO, 1 tablespoon
- ✓ Diced tomatoes, 2
- ✓ Sliced onion, 1

Directions:
- ❖ Place lentils in a bowl, cover with water and let stand for six hours.
- ❖ After six hours, drain the lentils completely.
- ❖ Place a bowl over normal heat. Place lentils and cover with fresh water. Allow to boil. Add turmeric. Lower heat and simmer until lentils are cooked.
- ❖ Remove from the pan and place in a bowl. Set aside.

Ingredients:
- ✓ Chopped garlic, 1 clove
- ✓ Grated ginger, 1 inch
- ✓ Turmeric, .5 tsp
- ✓ Cumin seeds, .5 tsp
- ✓ Chopped green peppers, 2
- ✓ Fine red lentils, 1 c.
- ❖ In another skillet over medium heat, heat the olive oil. Add the turmeric, cumin, ginger and onions. Cook until the onions are soft and the ginger is fragrant.
- ❖ Add the chiles and tomatoes and cook. Add the salt and cook for five minutes.
- ❖ Pour the lentil into this mixture and bring back to a simmer. As soon as it starts to cook, remove it from the hot temperature. Squeeze a little lemon
- ❖ Sprinkle with cilantro and serve with rice.

Nutrition: Calories

45)   Vegetables with wild rice

Preparation time: **Cooking time:**   Servings: 4

Ingredients:
- ✓ Halls
- ✓ Basil
- ✓ Cilantro
- ✓ Juice of a lime
- ✓ Chopped red bell pepper, 1
- ✓ Vegetable broth, .5 c.

Directions:
- ❖ Place all the chopped vegetables in a pan and add the vegetable broth.
- ❖ Steam fry the vegetables until cooked but still crispy.

Ingredients:
- ✓ Bean sprouts, 1 c.
- ✓ Chopped carrots, 2 c.
- ✓ Beans - green - diced, 1 c.
- ✓ Broccoli, cut, 1 c.
- ✓ Pak Choi, 1 c.
- ✓ Wild rice, 1 c.
- ❖ Using a mortar and pestle, grind the chili, basil, and cilantro until they form a paste. Add the lime juice and mix well.
- ❖ Place the rice on a serving plate. Add the vegetables on top and drizzle with the dressing.

Nutrition: Calories

46)   Spicy Lentil Soup

Preparation time: **Cooking time:**   Servings: 4

Ingredients:
- ✓ Halls
- ✓ Turmeric, .25 tsp
- ✓ Chopped garlic, 3 cloves
- ✓ Grated ginger, 1.5 inch piece
- ✓ Chopped tomato, 1

Directions:
- ❖ Place lentils in a colander and place under running water. Rinse until the soil and stones are released.
- ❖ Pour rinsed lentils into a pot. Add enough water to cover the lentils. Place the pot over medium heat and allow to boil.

Ingredients:
- ✓ Chopped Serrano chili pepper, 1
- ✓ Rinsed red lentils, 2 c.
- ✓ Topping:
- ✓ Coconut yogurt, .25 c.

- ❖ Lower the heat and simmer for ten minutes.
- ❖ Place the contents of the leftovers and then mix well to combine.
- ❖ Cook again until lentils are soft.
- ❖ Garnish with a spoonful of coconut yogurt.

Nutrition: Calories

47)   Leek soup with mushrooms

Preparation time: **Cooking time:**   **Servings: 4**

Ingredients:
- ✓ Sherry vinegar, 1.5 tablespoons
- ✓ Almond milk, .5 c.
- ✓ Cream of coconut, .66 c.
- ✓ Vegetable broth, 3 c.
- ✓ Chopped dill, 1 tablespoon
- ✓ Pepper
- ✓ Halls

Ingredients:
- ✓ Almond flour, 5 tablespoons
- ✓ Cleaned and sliced mushrooms, 7 c.
- ✓ Chopped garlic, 3 cloves
- ✓ Chopped leeks, 2.75 c.
- ✓ Vegetable oil, 3 tablespoons

Directions:
- ❖ Set a Dutch oven to medium and heat the oil. Add the leeks and bulb garlic and prepare until soft.
- ❖ Add the mushrooms, stir and cook for another 10 minutes.

- ❖ Add the salt, dill, pepper and flour. Mix well, until combined.
- ❖ Put the soup in and let it simmer. Reduce the heat and put in the rest of the ingredients. Stir well. Cook another ten minutes.
- ❖ Serve hot with almond flour bread.

Nutrition: Calories

48)   Fresh vegetarian pizza

Preparation time: **Cooking time:**   **Servings: 4**

Ingredients:
- Crust -
- ✓ Garlic bulb flavored powder, 0.5 teaspoon
- ✓ Sea salt, 0.5 teaspoon
- ✓ Coconut oil, 3 tablespoons
- ✓ Almond flour, 1.25 c.
- ✓ Tahini-Bee Spread -
- ✓ Pepper, pinch

Ingredients:
- ✓ Sea salt, a pinch
- ✓ Garlic, 2 cloves
- ✓ Lemon juice, one tablespoon
- ✓ Avocado oil, one tablespoon
- ✓ Middle Eastern Pasta, one tablespoon
- ✓ Peeled and diced beets, 2

Directions:
- ❖ Start by setting your oven to 375. Place some parchment on a tray.
- ❖ Mix together the salt, garlic powder, coconut oil and almond flour.
- ❖ Place it on the tray and squish it into a ball shape. Place another piece of parchment on top and roll out the dough into a 7x7 square. Bake for 14 minutes, or until it starts to brown.

- ❖ While the crust is cooking, add the pepper, salt, garlic, lemon juice, avocado oil, tahini, and beets to a food processor. Blend until creamy.
- ❖ To make your pizza, spread the crust with beet sauces and then top with your favorite alkaline friendly vegetables. Cut it into four and enjoy.

Nutrition: Calories

49)   Spicy Lentil Burger

Preparation time: **Cooking time:**   **Servings: 4**

Ingredients:
- ✓ Avocado oil, 1 tablespoon
- ✓ Coconut flour, 1 tablespoon
- ✓ Crushed garlic, 2 cloves
- ✓ Jalapeno cubes
- ✓ Chopped cilantro, .5 c.

Directions:
- ❖ Cook lentils according to package instructions and set aside to cool.
- ❖ Mix together the garlic, jalapeno, cilantro, onion, pepper, salt, almond meal and lentils until everything is well combined.
- ❖ Add half of the lentil mixture to a food processor and process until it reaches a paste-like consistency.
- ❖ Pour this into the bowl with the rest of the lentil mixture and toss to combine.

Ingredients:
- ✓ Diced onion, .5 c.
- ✓ Pepper, .5 tsp
- ✓ Sea salt, 0.5 teaspoons
- ✓ Almond flour, .5 c.
- ✓ Dried lentils, .5 c.
- ❖ The mixture will be very moist. Stir in the coconut flour to help get rid of the moisture and to help hold them together.
- ❖ Divide the mixture into quarters. Squeeze a quarter of the mixture between your hands to flatten it into a hamburger shape. Do this for the remaining three sections.
- ❖ Heat the oil in a large skillet and place the burgers in it. Prepare the burgers 4 to 6 minutes on both sides, or until golden brown. When you flip them, do so carefully so they don't fall apart. Enjoy.

Nutrition: Calories

50)   Roasted cauliflower rolls

Preparation time: **Cooking time:**   **Servings: 2**

Ingredients:
- ✓ Cauliflower -
- ✓ Pepper, .25 tsp
- ✓ Sea salt, .25 tsp
- ✓ Garlic powder, .5 tsp
- ✓ Nutritional yeast, .25 c.
- ✓ Almond flour, .25 c.
- ✓ Avocado oil, 1 tablespoon
- ✓ Bitten cauliflower florets, 2 c.
- ✓ Sauce -
- ✓ Sea Salt

Ingredients:
- ✓ Apple cider vinegar, 2 tablespoons
- ✓ Garlic, 2 cloves
- ✓ Habanero Pepper
- ✓ Mango cubes, 1 c.
- ✓ Assembly -
- ✓ Canola shoots, 2 leaves
- ✓ Mixed salad, 1 c.

Directions:
- ❖ Start by setting your kitchen appliance to three hundred and fifty degrees then place paper on a kitchen wrap.
- ❖ To prepare the cauliflower, toss it in the avocado oil and make sure it's evenly coated.
- ❖ In a container, combine together all the seasonings: pepper, salt, garlic powder, healthy mushrooms, along with almond flour.
- ❖ Sprinkle breading over cauliflower and toss, making sure cauliflower is well coated. Spread on the baking sheet.

- ❖ Bake thirty to thirty-five minutes, or until cauliflower is soft.
- ❖ While the cauliflower is cooking, add the salt, vinegar, garlic, habanero and mango to your blender and blend until well combined. Be sure to use gloves or wash your hands thoroughly when you need to handle the habanero.
- ❖ To assemble, divide the salad mix between the collard leaves, top with the cauliflower and pour the sauce over it. Wrap the whole thing like a burrito and enjoy.

Nutrition: Calories

51)   Sliced sweet potato with artichoke cream and peppers

Preparation time: **Cooking time:**   **Servings: 4**

Ingredients:
- ✓ Pepper, .25 tsp
- ✓ Salt, .5 tsp
- ✓ Avocado oil, 6 tablespoons - divided
- ✓ Red bell pepper cut into quarters

Directions:
- ❖ Start by setting the oven to 350. Place parchment on a tray and set aside.
- ❖ Spread the bell bell pepper and sweet potato on the sheet tray and top with two teaspoons of avocado oil, a pinch of pepper and a pinch of salt.

Ingredients:
- ✓ Unpeeled sweet potatoes, 2 cut into 4 slices lengthwise
- ✓ Garlic, 2 cloves
- ✓ Artichoke hearts, 14 oz can

- ❖ Bake for 30 minutes. Turn them over and bake for another 15 minutes.
- ❖ Add the roasted red bell pepper to a food processor along with the garlic, artichoke hearts, pepper, salt and remaining avocado oil. Pulse until combined but still somewhat chunky. Adjust seasonings as needed.
- ❖ Top the sweet potato slices with the cream and enjoy.

Nutrition: Calories

52)   Cooking scallops, onions and potatoes

Preparation time:	Cooking time:	Servings: 4

Ingredients:

- ✓ Cashew cheese sauce -
- ✓ Sea salt, 0.5 teaspoons
- ✓ Nutritional yeast, .5 c.
- ✓ Almond milk, 1 c.
- ✓ Raw cashews, 1 c.
- ✓ Scallop Bake -
- ✓ Chopped tarragon, 1 tablespoon

Directions:

- ❖ To make the cheese sauce, add the cashews to a bowl and cover them with room temperature water. Let them soak for 15-20 minutes and then drain and rinse them.
- ❖ Blend together cashews with remaining cheese sauce ingredients until smooth and creamy. Set aside until later.
- ❖ Start by heating the oven to 375.
- ❖ Combine the onions and potatoes in a bowl with the avocado oil. Add the tarragon, pepper and salt, making sure everything is well coated.

Nutrition: Calories

Ingredients:

- ✓ Pepper, 1 teaspoon
- ✓ Sea salt, one teaspoon
- ✓ Oil - Avocado, one tablespoon
- ✓ Chopped small onion bulbs, 1.5
- ✓ New potatoes, thinly sliced, 8

- ❖ Using an 8-inch square baking dish, place the potato and onion mixture in the dish. Do your best to arrange them in nice rows. It doesn't have to be perfect.
- ❖ Bake for 45 minutes, or until potatoes are soft
- ❖ Remove from oven and top with cheese sauce. Divide among four plates and enjoy. You can also slide this on, and bake inside the cooking appliance on about 5 minutes in order to warm the cheese sauce through before serving.

53)   Spicy cilantro and coconut soup

Preparation time:	Cooking time:	Servings: 2

Ingredients:

- ✓ Cilantro leaves, 2 tablespoons
- ✓ Jalapeno
- ✓ Lime juice, 1 tablespoon
- ✓ Whole Coconut Milk, 13.5 oz. can

Directions:

- ❖ Add the avocado oil to a medium skillet and heat. Add the salt, garlic and onion, cooking three to five minutes, or until the onion bulbs become smooth.

Nutrition: Calories

Ingredients:

- ✓ Sea salt, .25 tsp
- ✓ Crushed garlic, 3 cloves
- ✓ Diced onion, .5 c.
- ✓ Avocado oil, 2 tablespoons
- ❖ Place the onion mixture, cilantro, jalapeno, lime juice and coconut milk in a blender and blend until creamy.
- ❖ Pour into a bowl and enjoy.

54)   Tarragon soup

Preparation time:	Cooking time:	Servings: 2

Ingredients:

- ✓ Chopped fresh tarragon, 2 tablespoons
- ✓ Celery stalk
- ✓ Raw cashews, .5 c.
- ✓ Lemon juice, 1 tablespoon
- ✓ Whole Coconut Milk, 13.5 oz. can

Directions:

- ❖ Add the oil to a medium skillet and heat it up. Put all the seasonings: pepper, salt, garlic bulbs, along with the onion bulbs then prepare about three to five minutes, or until the onions become soft.

Nutrition: Calories

Ingredients:

- ✓ Pepper, .5 tsp - divided
- ✓ Sea Salt, .5 tsp - divided
- ✓ Crushed garlic, 3 cloves
- ✓ Diced onion, .5 c.
- ✓ Avocado oil, 1 tablespoon
- ❖ Using a high-speed blender, add the onion mixture, tarragon, celery, cashews, lemon juice, and coconut milk. Blend until smooth. Taste and adjust seasonings if necessary.
- ❖ Divide between two bowls and enjoy. You can also add back into a pot and reheat before serving.

55)   Asparagus and artichoke soup

Preparation time: **Cooking time:**   **Servings: 4**

Ingredients:

- ✓ Artichoke hearts halved and chopped, 1 can
- ✓ Almond milk, 2 c.
- ✓ Pepper, .5 tsp
- ✓ Sea Salt, .5 - .75 tsp
- ✓ Vegetable broth, 2 c.
- ✓ Asparagus diced, 8 stalks

Directions:

- ❖ Add the garlic, avocado oil and onion to a skillet and cook for a few minutes, or until the onion bulbs have softened and weakened.
- ❖ Place the cooked vegetables in a pot and add the pepper, salt, vegetable stock, asparagus and potatoes. Stir everything together and let it simmer. Lower the heat and simmer gently eighteen to twenty minutes, or until the potatoes have become soft.

Nutrition: Calories

Ingredients:

- ✓ Cubed potatoes, 1 c.
- ✓ Crushed garlic, 2 cloves
- ✓ Avocado oil, 1 tablespoon
- ✓ Diced onion, .5 c.

- ❖ Add a little more broth if you need it, so that the liquid remains about an inch above the vegetables.
- ❖ Set the pot away from the heat and let it cool.
- ❖ Using a blender, blend the cooled soup with the artichokes and almond milk until everything is well combined and smooth. Adjust seasonings as needed. You can add more broth or milk to thicken everything if needed.
- ❖ Pour back into the pot and allow to heat over low heat until ready to serve.

56)   Mint and berry soup

Preparation time: **Cooking time:**   **Servings: 1**

Ingredients:

- ✓ Sweetener -
- ✓ Water, .25 c - more if needed
- ✓ Unrefined whole cane sugar, .25 c.
-    Soup -
- ✓ Water, .5 c.

Directions:

- ❖ Add the water and sugar to a small saucepan and cook, stirring constantly, until the sugar has dissolved. Allow to cool.
- ❖ Add the mint leaves, lemon juice, water, berries and cooled sugar mixture to a blender. Blend everything until smooth.

Nutrition: Calories

Ingredients:

- ✓ Mixed berries, 1 c.
- ✓ Mint leaves, 8
- ✓ Lemon juice, 1 teaspoon

- ❖ Pour into a bowl and then refrigerate until the broth is completely cooled. This will take about 20 minutes.
- ❖ Enjoy.

57)   Mushroom soup

Preparation time: **Cooking time:**   **Servings: 2**

Ingredients:

- ✓ Whole Coconut Milk, 13.5 oz. can
- ✓ Vegetable stock, 1 c.
- ✓ Pepper, .5 tsp
- ✓ Sea salt, .75 tsp
- ✓ Crush the garlic clove
- ✓ Diced onion, 1 cup

Directions:

- ❖ Heat the fat in a very massive pan, then put all the seasonings: pepper, salt, garlic, onion bulb and mushrooms. Boil and prepare for a few minutes, or until onions are soft.
- ❖ Stir in the coconut amino acid, thyme, coconut milk and vegetable broth.

Nutrition: Calories

Ingredients:

- ✓ Cut cremini mushrooms, 1 cup
- ✓ Chinese black mushrooms cut into pieces, one cup
- ✓ Avocado oil, 1 tablespoon
- ✓ Coconut amino acids, 1 tablespoon
- ✓ Dried thyme, .5 tsp

- ❖ Lower the heat and let the broth simmer for about fifteen minutes. Stir the broth occasionally.
- ❖ Taste and adjust seasoning as needed. Divide between two bowls and enjoy.

58) Potato and lentil stew

Preparation time: **Cooking time:**   **Servings: 4**

Ingredients:

- ✓ Chopped oregano sprigs, 2 sprigs
- ✓ Diced celery stalk
- ✓ Potato diced and peeled, 1 c.
- ✓ Sliced carrots, 2
- ✓ Dried lentils, 1 c.
- ✓ Spicy seasoning / Pepper, one teaspoon
- ✓ Sea salt, one to 1.5 teaspoons

Directions:

- ❖ Using a large cooking utensil, heat the avocado fat along with the inclusion of seasonings: pepper, salt, garlic bulbs, along with the onion. Cook three to five minutes, or until onion is soft.
- ❖ Add the tarragon, oregano, celery, potato, carrots, lentils and 2 ½ cups of vegetable stock. Stir everything together.

Ingredients:

- ✓ Crushed garlic bulbs, two buds
- ✓ Diced onion, .5 c.
- ✓ Avocado oil, 2 tablespoons
- ✓ Whole Coconut Milk, 13.5 oz. can
- ✓ Vegetable broth, 5 c - divided
- ✓ Chopped tarragon, 2 sprigs

- ❖ Allow the saucepan to heat back up and then lower the heat. Allow to cook, stirring frequently. Add more vegetable broth in half-cup portions, if necessary, to make sure the lentils have enough liquid to cook. Let the stew cook for 20-25 minutes, or until the lentils and potatoes are soft.
- ❖ Remove stew from heat and stir in coconut milk. Divide among four bowls and enjoy.

Nutrition: Calories

59) Mixed mushroom stew

Preparation time: 15 minutes   **Cooking time**: 15 minutes   **Servings: 4**

Ingredients:

- ✓ 2 tablespoons of olive oil
- ✓ 2 onions, chopped
- ✓ 3 garlic cloves, minced
- ✓ ½ pound fresh mushrooms, chopped
- ✓ ¼ pound fresh shiitake mushrooms, chopped

Directions:

- ❖ In a large skillet, heat the oil over medium heat and sauté the onion and garlic for 4-5 minutes.
- ❖ Add the mushrooms, salt and black pepper and cook for 4-5 minutes.

Ingredients:

- ✓ ¼ pound fresh Portobello mushrooms, chopped
- ✓ Sea salt and freshly ground black pepper, to taste
- ✓ ¼ cup homemade vegetable broth
- ✓ ½ cup unsweetened coconut milk
- ✓ 2 tablespoons fresh parsley, chopped
- ❖ Add the broth and coconut milk and bring to a gentle boil.
- ❖ Simmer for 4-5 minutes or until desired doneness.
- ❖ Add the parsley and remove from heat.
- ❖ Serve warm.

Nutrition: Calories

60) Mixed stew of spicy vegetables

Preparation time: 20 minutes   **Cooking time**: 35 minutes   **Servings: 8**

Ingredients:

- ✓ 2 tablespoons of coconut oil
- ✓ 1 large sweet onion, chopped
- ✓ 1 medium parsnip, peeled and chopped
- ✓ 3 tablespoons of homemade tomato paste
- ✓ 2 large garlic cloves, minced
- ✓ ½ teaspoon of cinnamon powder
- ✓ ½ teaspoon ground ginger
- ✓ 1 teaspoon of ground cumin
- ✓ ¼ teaspoon cayenne pepper

Directions:

- ❖ In a large soup pot, melt the coconut oil over medium-high heat and sauté the onion for about 5 minutes.
- ❖ Add the parsnips and sauté for about 3 minutes.
- ❖ Add the tomato paste, garlic and spices and sauté for 2 minutes.

Ingredients:

- ✓ 2 medium carrots, peeled and chopped
- ✓ 2 medium purple potatoes, peeled and cut into pieces
- ✓ 2 medium sweet potatoes, peeled and cut into pieces
- ✓ 4 cups of homemade vegetable broth
- ✓ 2 tablespoons fresh lemon juice
- ✓ 2 cups fresh cabbage, hard ribs removed and chopped
- ✓ ¼ cup fresh parsley leaves, chopped

- ❖ Stir in the carrots, potatoes, sweet potatoes and broth and bring to a boil.
- ❖ Reduce heat to medium-low and simmer, covered for about 20 minutes.
- ❖ Add the lemon juice and cabbage and simmer for 5 minutes.
- ❖ Serve with a garnish of parsley.

Nutrition: Calories

Alkaline Diet Snack Recipes

61)　Bean burgers

Preparation time: 20 minutes

Cooking time: 25 minutes

Servings: 8

Ingredients:
- ✓ ½ cup of walnuts
- ✓ 1 carrot, peeled and chopped
- ✓ 1 celery stalk, chopped
- ✓ 4 shallots, chopped
- ✓ 5 cloves of garlic, minced

Directions:
- ❖ Preheat oven to 400 degrees F. Line a baking sheet with baking paper.
- ❖ In a food processor, add the walnuts and pulse until finely ground.
- ❖ Add the carrot, celery, shallot and garlic and run through a meat grinder until finely chopped.
- ❖ Transfer the vegetable mixture to a large bowl.
- ❖ In the same food processor, add the beans and pulse until chopped.

Ingredients:
- ✓ 2¼ cups canned black beans, rinsed and drained
- ✓ 2½ cups sweet potato, peeled and grated
- ✓ ½ teaspoon of red pepper flakes, crushed
- ✓ ¼ teaspoon cayenne pepper
- ✓ Sea salt and freshly ground black pepper, to taste
- ❖ Add 1 1/2 cups sweet potatoes and pulse until a chunky mixture forms.
- ❖ Transfer the bean mixture to the bowl with the vegetable mixture.
- ❖ Stir in remaining sweet potato and spices and mix until well combined.
- ❖ Make 8 equal-sized patties from the dough.
- ❖ Arrange the meatballs on the prepared baking sheet in a single layer.
- ❖ Bake for about 25 minutes.
- ❖ Serve hot.

Nutrition: Calories

62)　Grilled watermelon

Preparation time: 10 minutes

Cooking time: 4 minutes

Servings: 4

Ingredients:
- ✓ 1 watermelon, peeled and cut into 1 inch thick wedges
- ✓ 1 garlic clove, finely chopped
- ✓ 2 tablespoons fresh lime juice

Directions:
- ❖ Preheat the grill to high heat. Grease the grill grate.
- ❖ Grill the watermelon pieces for about 2 minutes on both sides.

Ingredients:
- ✓ Pinch of cayenne pepper
- ✓ Pinch of sea salt

- ❖ Meanwhile, in a small bowl mix together the remaining ingredients.
- ❖ Drizzle the watermelon slices with the lemon mixture and serve.

Nutrition: Calories

63)　Mango sauce

Preparation time: 15 minutes

Cooking time:

Servings: 6

Ingredients:
- ✓ 1 avocado, peeled, pitted and cut into cubes
- ✓ 2 tablespoons fresh lime juice
- ✓ 1 mango, peeled, pitted and cut into cubes
- ✓ 1 cup cherry tomatoes, halved

Directions:
- ❖ In a large bowl, add the avocado and lime juice and mix well.

Ingredients:
- ✓ 1 jalapeño bell pepper, seeded and chopped
- ✓ 1 tablespoon fresh cilantro, chopped
- ✓ Sea salt, to taste

- ❖ Add remaining ingredients and stir to combine.
- ❖ Serve immediately.

Nutrition: Calories

64)　Avocado gazpacho

Preparation time: 15 minutes

Cooking time:

Servings: 6

Ingredients:
- ✓ 3 large avocados, peeled, pitted and chopped
- ✓ 1/3 cup fresh coriander leaves
- ✓ 3 cups of homemade vegetable broth
- ✓ 2 tablespoons fresh lemon juice

Directions:
- ❖ Add all ingredients to a high speed blender and pulse until smooth.

Ingredients:
- ✓ 1 teaspoon of ground cumin
- ✓ ¼ teaspoon cayenne pepper
- ✓ Sea salt, to taste

- ❖ Transfer the soup to a large bowl.
- ❖ Cover the bowl and refrigerate to chill for at least 2-3 hours before serving.

65)   Roasted chickpeas

Preparation time: 10 minutes   **Cooking time**: 45 minutes   **Servings: 12**

Ingredients:
- ✓   4 cups of cooked chickpeas
- ✓   2 garlic cloves, minced
- ✓   ½ teaspoon dried oregano, crushed
- ✓   ½ teaspoon of smoked paprika

Ingredients:
- ✓   ¼ teaspoon ground cumin
- ✓   Sea salt, to taste
- ✓   1 tablespoon of olive oil

Directions:
- ❖   Preheat oven to 400 degrees F. Grease a large baking sheet.
- ❖   Arrange the chickpeas on the prepared baking sheet in a single layer.
- ❖   Roast for about 30 minutes, stirring the chickpeas every 10 minutes.
- ❖   Meanwhile, in a small bowl, mix together garlic, thyme and spices.

- ❖   Remove the baking sheet from the oven.
- ❖   Pour the garlic mixture and oil over the chickpeas and toss to coat well.
- ❖   Roast for another 10-15 minutes or so.
- ❖   Now, turn off the oven but let the pan sit for about 10 minutes before serving.

Nutrition: Calories

66)   Banana chips

Preparation time: 10 minutes   **Cooking time**: 1 hour and 10 minutes   **Portions:**

Ingredients:
- ✓   2 large bananas, peeled and cut into ¼ inch thick slices

Ingredients:

Directions:
- ❖   Prepare oven for 250 degrees F. Line a large baking sheet with baking paper.

- ❖   Arrange the banana slices on the prepared baking sheet in a single layer.
- ❖   Bake for about 1 hour.

Nutrition: Calories

67)   Roasted cashews

Preparation time: 10 minutes   **Cooking time**: 10 minutes   **Servings: 12**

Ingredients:
- ✓   2 cups of raw cashews
- ✓   ½ teaspoon of ground cumin
- ✓   ¼ teaspoon cayenne pepper

Ingredients:
- ✓   Pinch of salt
- ✓   1 tablespoon fresh lemon juice

Directions:
- ❖   Preheat oven to 400 degrees F. Line a large baking sheet with a piece of foil.
- ❖   In a large bowl, add the cashews and spices and stir to coat well.

- ❖   Transfer cashews to the prepared baking dish.
- ❖   Roast for about 8-10 minutes.
- ❖   Drizzle with lemon juice and serve.

Nutrition: Calories

68)   Dried orange slices

Preparation time: 10 minutes   **Cooking time**: 1 hour   **Servings: 15**

Ingredients:
- ✓   4 navel oranges without seeds, cut into thin slices (DO NOT peel the oranges)

Ingredients:

Directions:
- ❖   Set the dehydrator to 135 degrees F.

- ❖   Arrange the orange slices on the sheets of the dehydrator.
- ❖   Dehydrate for about 10 hours.

Nutrition: Calories

69)   Chickpea hummus

Preparation time: 10 minutes   **Cooking time**:   **Servings: 12**

Ingredients:
- ✓ 2 (15-ounce) cans of chickpeas, rinsed and drained
- ✓ ½ cup of tahini
- ✓ 1 garlic clove, minced
- ✓ 2 tablespoons fresh lemon juice

Directions:
- ❖ In a blender, add all ingredients and pulse until smooth.

Ingredients:
- ✓ Sea salt, to taste
- ✓ Filtered water, if necessary
- ✓ 1 tablespoon olive oil plus more for spraying
- ✓ Pinch of cayenne pepper
- ❖ Transfer hummus to a large bowl and drizzle with oil.
- ❖ Sprinkle with cayenne pepper and serve immediately.

Nutrition: Calories

70)   Avocado chips in the oven

Preparation time: 7 minutes   **Cooking time**: 17 minutes   **Servings: 4**

Ingredients:
- ✓ ½ cup of almond flour
- ✓ ½ teaspoon ground paprika, plus more for dusting
- ✓ 2 tablespoons of nutritional yeast
- ✓ ½ teaspoon of garlic powder

Directions:
- ❖ Preheat the oven to 420°F.
- ❖ In a small bowl, mix together the almond flour, nutritional yeast, garlic powder, paprika and salt until well combined.
- ❖ Halve and pit the avocados, and split each half from pole to pole. Remove the skin.
- ❖ Add the almond milk to another small bowl.
- ❖ Line a baking sheet with baking paper.

Ingredients:
- ✓ 2 avocados, slightly unripe
- ✓ ½ cup of almond milk
- ✓ ½ teaspoon of sea salt

- ❖ Dip an avocado slice first in the milk and then in the coating mixture, turning it gently to make sure it is completely covered, and place it on the prepared baking sheet. Repeat with the other avocado slices.
- ❖ Bake for 15-17 minutes, being careful not to overcook or burn them.
- ❖ Remove from oven, sprinkle with more paprika and serve immediately.

Nutrition: Calories

71)   Dried apples with cinnamon

Preparation time: 3 minutes   **Cooking time**: 3 hours   **Servings: 1**

Ingredients:
- ✓ 2 apples, sliced
- ✓ 1 teaspoon ground cinnamon

Directions:
- ❖ Spread all the apple slices on a baking sheet.
- ❖ Cough up the slices with cinnamon and olive oil.

Ingredients:
- ✓ 1 teaspoon of olive oil

- ❖ Bake for 3 hours at 200 degrees F.
- ❖ Serve and enjoy!

Nutrition: Calories

72)   Guacamole sauce

Preparation time: 5 minutes   **Cooking time**:   **Servings: 1**

Ingredients:
- ✓ ½ cup sauce,
- ✓ 2 crushed avocados,

Directions:
- ❖ Mix all ingredients together in a bowl.

Ingredients:
- ✓ 2 tablespoons of chopped coriander
- ✓ Salt, to taste

- ❖ Serve and enjoy!

Nutrition: Calories

73)   Apple chip

Preparation time: 3 minutes

Cooking time: 40 minutes

Servings: 2

Ingredients:

- ✓   2 apples, core and thin slices
- ✓   2 tbsp white sugar

Ingredients:

- ✓   ½ teaspoon ground cinnamon

Directions:

- ❖   Preheat the oven to 225 degrees F.
- ❖   Place the apple slices on a baking sheet.

- ❖   Sprinkle with cinnamon and sugar.
- ❖   Bake for 40 minutes and then serve.

Nutrition: Calories

74)   Alka-Goulash fast

Preparation time: 10 minutes

Cooking time: 15 minutes

Servings: 4

Ingredients:

- ✓   1 onion, finely chopped
- ✓   1 garlic clove, crushed
- ✓   2 carrots, diced
- ✓   3 zucchini, diced
- ✓   2 tablespoons of olive oil
- ✓   1 tablespoon of paprika
- ✓   ¼ teaspoon ground nutmeg

Ingredients:

- ✓   1 tablespoon fresh parsley, chopped
- ✓   1 tablespoon of tomato puree
- ✓   2 cups of tomatoes, peeled
- ✓   2 cups of cooked, drained and rinsed red beans
- ✓   ½ cup of tomato juice
- ✓   Salt and black pepper to taste

Directions:

- ❖   Sauté onion, garlic, carrot and zucchini in olive oil over medium heat for 5 minutes until softened.
- ❖   Add the paprika, nutmeg, parsley and tomato puree.

- ❖   Add the tomatoes, red beans and tomato juice and stir.
- ❖   Simmer for 10 minutes until heated through.
- ❖   Serve immediately. Enjoy!

Nutrition: Calories

75)   Eggplant Caviar

Preparation time:

Cooking time:

Servings: 2-4

Ingredients:

- ✓   2 medium eggplants
- ✓   2 tablespoons of olive oil
- ✓   1 onion, finely chopped
- ✓   1 green bell pepper, seedless and finely chopped
- ✓   2 spoons of tomato puree

Ingredients:

- ✓   4 tablespoons of water
- ✓   2 tablespoons of lemon juice
- ✓   Salt and black pepper to taste
- ✓   Gluten-free bread or wrap of your choice

Directions:

- ❖   Pierce eggplant several times with a sharp knife. Boil or steam until soft. Allow them to cool.
- ❖   Remove stems and scoop out pulp from eggplant. Finely chop the soft pulp.
- ❖   Add the olive oil to a large skillet over medium heat. Sauté the onion and green bell pepper until the onion is translucent.
- ❖   Add the eggplant, tomato puree, water, salt and black pepper to the skillet.

- ❖   Reduce the heat and cook over low heat. Stir frequently for 20-30 minutes, at which point the mixture will begin to thicken.
- ❖   Place the mixture in a bowl and stir in the lemon juice.
- ❖   Allow the mixture to cool and place in the refrigerator.
- ❖   Serve cold with a slice of gluten-free bread, a wrap, or chopped vegetables (e.g., carrots or cucumbers).

Nutrition: Calories

76) Spiced nut mixture

Preparation time: **Cooking time:**   **Servings: 4**

Ingredients:

- ✓ 1/3 cup sesame seeds
- ✓ 1/2 cup hazelnuts, blanched
- ✓ 3 tablespoons of coriander seeds
- ✓ 2 tablespoons of cumin seeds

Directions:

- ❖ Dry-fry sesame seeds in a large skillet over medium heat until golden brown. Remove from heat and let cool in a bowl.
- ❖ Toast the hazelnuts in the same pan until shiny and starting to turn golden brown. Add to the sesame seeds and let cool.
- ❖ Dry fry the coriander and cumin seeds until fragrant, but be sure not to let them burn. Add them to the bowl of nuts and sesame seeds and let cool.

Nutrition: Calories

Ingredients:

- ✓ Hot gluten-free tortillas of your choice, cut into strips or chopped vegetables
- ✓ Olive Oil
- ✓ 1/2 teaspoon salt
- ✓ Black pepper to taste
- ❖ Now place the mixture in a food processor and add salt and black pepper to taste. Process the mixture until it reaches the consistency of a coarse, dry powder.
- ❖ Serve with gluten-free tortilla wraps or veggies alongside a bowl of olive oil. To consume, dip the bread or raw veggies, into the oil and then into the spicy nut mixture.

77) Garlic mushrooms

Preparation time: **Cooking time:**   **Servings: 4**

Ingredients:

- ✓ 2 tablespoons of olive oil
- ✓ 2 garlic cloves, crushed
- ✓ 1/4 teaspoon of dried thyme
- ✓ 1/4 teaspoon of dried parsley
- ✓ 1/4 teaspoon of dried sage
- ✓ 2 cups of mushrooms, cut in quarters

Directions:

- ❖ Sauté garlic in olive oil until softened and beginning to brown.
- ❖ Add the dried herbs and mushrooms and season with salt and black pepper to taste.

Nutrition: Calories

Ingredients:

- ✓ Chopped raw vegetables of your choice (e.g. cucumbers, carrots, peppers)
- ✓ 2 tablespoons chives, chopped
- ✓ Salt and black pepper to taste

- ❖ Sauté this mixture over low heat for about 10 minutes, until the mushrooms are soft.
- ❖ Serve the mushrooms alongside the raw vegetables. Garnish with the chopped chives.
- ❖ Enjoy!

78) Hummus

Preparation time: **Cooking time:**   **Portions:**

Ingredients:

- ✓ 1 cup cooked chickpeas, stock reserve
- ✓ 4 tablespoons of light tahini
- ✓ Juice of 2 lemons

Directions:

- ❖ Blend chickpeas with 1/8 cup reserved broth from cooking.
- ❖ Add the lemon juice, garlic, tahini and half of the olive oil.
- ❖ Blend this mixture until smooth.

Nutrition: Calories

Ingredients:

- ✓ 6 tablespoons of olive oil
- ✓ 4 garlic cloves, crushed
- ✓ Salt to taste
- ❖ Allow to rest for about an hour before serving.
- ❖ To serve, drizzle the remaining olive oil over each individual serving. Serve alongside some raw vegetables.

79)   Paleo vegan zucchini hummus

Preparation time: Cooking time: Portions:

Ingredients:
- ✓   1 cup sliced zucchini
- ✓   4 tablespoons of light tahini
- ✓   Juice of 2 lemons

Directions:
- ❖   Combine zucchini, lemon juice, garlic, tahini and half of the olive oil in a blender.
- ❖   Blend this mixture until smooth.

Nutrition: Calories

Ingredients:
- ✓   6 tablespoons of olive oil
- ✓   4 garlic cloves, crushed
- ✓   Himalayan salt to taste
- ❖   Allow to rest for about an hour before serving.
- ❖   To serve, drizzle the remaining olive oil over each individual serving. Serve alongside some raw vegetables or sprouted bread.

80)   German style sweet potato salad

Preparation time: Cooking time: Servings: 2-4

Ingredients:
- ✓   2 cups sweet potatoes, chopped
- ✓   1 cup baby spinach
- ✓   1 cup of cherry tomatoes
- ✓   1 red bell pepper
- ✓   4 tablespoons of olive oil

Directions:
- ❖   Clean and peel the potatoes. Boil them in a saucepan until tender. The time required will vary depending on their size.
- ❖   Meanwhile, sauté the garlic and scallions in a skillet over medium heat for 2-3 minutes, until slightly soft.
- ❖   Add the dill and sauté for about 1 minute.

Nutrition: Calories

Ingredients:
- ✓   4 shallots, cut and finely chopped
- ✓   1 garlic clove, crushed or minced
- ✓   2 tablespoons fresh dill, finely chopped
- ✓   2 tablespoons fresh parsley, chopped
- ✓   Salt and black pepper to taste
- ❖   Remove from heat and season to taste with salt and black pepper.
- ❖   Drain the potatoes once they are cooked, and pour the herb dressing over them while they are hot.
- ❖   Let cool and then add the rest of the ingredients and garnish with parsley. Serve fresh!

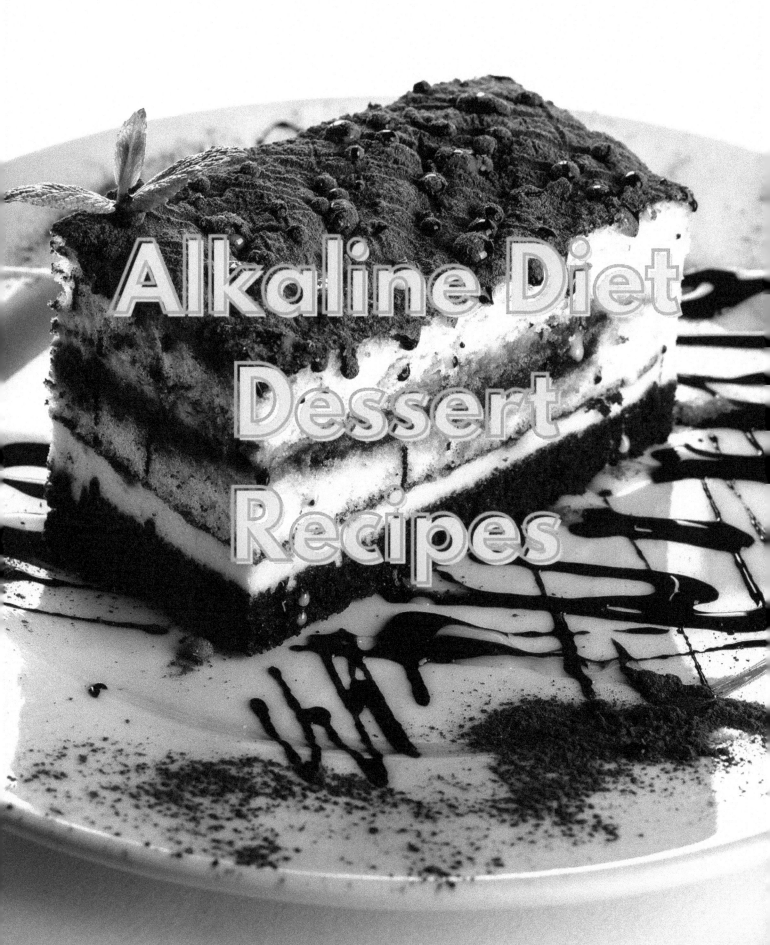

81)   Red fruit and vegetable smoothie

Preparation time: 10 minutes   **Cooking time**:   **Servings**: 2

Ingredients:
- ✓ ½ cup fresh raspberries
- ✓ ½ cup fresh strawberries
- ✓ ½ red bell pepper, seeded and chopped
- ✓ ½ cup red cabbage, chopped

Directions:
- ❖ Place all ingredients in a high speed blender and pulse until creamy.

Nutrition: Calories

Ingredients:
- ✓ 1 small tomato
- ✓ 1 cup of water
- ✓ ½ cup of ice cubes

- ❖ Pour the smoothie into two glasses and serve immediately.

82)   Kale Smoothie

Preparation time: 10 minutes   **Cooking time**:   **Servings**: 2

Ingredients:
- ✓ 3 fresh cabbage stalks, cut and chopped
- ✓ 1-2 celery stalks, chopped
- ✓ ½ avocado, peeled, pitted and chopped

Directions:
- ❖ Place all ingredients in a high speed blender and pulse until creamy.

Nutrition: Calories

Ingredients:
- ✓ ½ inch ginger root, chopped
- ✓ ½ inch turmeric root, chopped
- ✓ 2 cups of coconut milk
- ❖ Pour the smoothie into two glasses and serve immediately.

83)   Green Tofu Smoothie

Preparation time: 10 minutes   **Cooking time**:   **Servings**: 2

Ingredients:
- ✓ 1½ cups cucumber, peeled and coarsely chopped
- ✓ 3 cups fresh spinach
- ✓ 2 cups of frozen broccoli
- ✓ ½ cup silken tofu, drained and pressed

Directions:
- ❖ Place all ingredients in a high speed blender and pulse until creamy.

Nutrition: Calories

Ingredients:
- ✓ 1 tablespoon fresh lime juice
- ✓ 4-5 drops of liquid stevia
- ✓ 1 cup unsweetened almond milk
- ✓ ½ cup ice, crushed
- ❖ Pour the smoothie into two glasses and serve immediately.

84)   Grape and chard smoothie

Preparation time: 10 minutes   **Cooking time**:   **Servings**: 2

Ingredients:
- ✓ 2 cups of green grapes without seeds
- ✓ 2 cups fresh beets, cut and chopped
- ✓ 2 tablespoons of maple syrup

Directions:
- ❖ Place all ingredients in a high speed blender and pulse until creamy.

Nutrition: Calories

Ingredients:
- ✓ 1 teaspoon fresh lemon juice
- ✓ 1½ cups of water
- ✓ 4 ice cubes
- ❖ Pour the smoothie into two glasses and serve immediately.

85)   Matcha Smoothie

Preparation time: 10 minutes   Cooking time: Servings: 2

Ingredients:
- ✓ 2 tablespoons of chia seeds
- ✓ 2 teaspoons of matcha green tea powder
- ✓ ½ teaspoon fresh lemon juice
- ✓ ½ teaspoon xanthan gum

Directions:
- ❖ Place all ingredients in a high speed blender and pulse until creamy.

Nutrition: Calories

Ingredients:
- ✓ 8-10 drops of liquid stevia
- ✓ 4 tablespoons of coconut cream
- ✓ 1½ cups unsweetened almond milk
- ✓ ¼ cup ice cubes
- ❖ Pour the smoothie into two glasses and serve immediately.

86)   Banana Smoothie

Preparation time: 10 minutes   Cooking time: Servings: 2

Ingredients:
- ✓ 2 cups of cooled unsweetened almond milk
- ✓ 1 large frozen banana, peeled and sliced

Directions:
- ❖ Place all ingredients in a high speed blender and pulse until creamy.

Nutrition: Calories

Ingredients:
- ✓ 1 tablespoon almonds, chopped
- ✓ 1 teaspoon of organic vanilla extract
- ❖ Pour the smoothie into two glasses and serve immediately.

87)   Strawberry Smoothie

Preparation time: 10 minutes   Cooking time: Servings: 2

Ingredients:
- ✓ 2 cups of cooled unsweetened almond milk
- ✓ 1½ cups of frozen strawberries

Directions:
- ❖ Add all ingredients to a high speed blender and pulse until smooth.

Nutrition: Calories

Ingredients:
- ✓ 1 banana, peeled and sliced
- ✓ ¼ teaspoon of organic vanilla extract
- ❖ Pour the smoothie into two glasses and serve immediately.

88)   Raspberry and tofu smoothie

Preparation time: 15 minutes   Cooking time: Servings: 2

Ingredients:
- ✓ 1½ cups of fresh raspberries
- ✓ 6 ounces of firm silken tofu, drained
- ✓ 1/8 teaspoon of coconut extract

Directions:
- ❖ Add all ingredients to a high speed blender and pulse until smooth.

Nutrition: Calories

Ingredients:
- ✓ 1 teaspoon of stevia powder
- ✓ 1½ cups unsweetened almond milk
- ✓ ¼ cup ice cubes, crushed
- ❖ Pour the smoothie into two glasses and serve immediately.

89)   Mango Smoothie

Preparation time: 10 minutes   **Cooking time**:   **Servings**: 2

Ingredients:
- ✓ 2 cups frozen mango, peeled, pitted and chopped
- ✓ ¼ cup almond butter
- ✓ Pinch of ground turmeric

Directions:
- ❖ Add all ingredients to a high speed blender and pulse until smooth.

Nutrition: Calories

Ingredients:
- ✓ 2 tablespoons fresh lemon juice
- ✓ 1¼ cup unsweetened almond milk
- ✓ ¼ cup ice cubes
- ❖ Pour the smoothie into two glasses and serve immediately.

90)   Pineapple Smoothie

Preparation time: 10 minutes   **Cooking time**:   **Servings**: 2

Ingredients:
- ✓ 2 cups pineapple, chopped
- ✓ ½ teaspoon fresh ginger, peeled and chopped
- ✓ ½ teaspoon ground turmeric
- ✓ 1 teaspoon of natural immune support supplement*.

Directions:
- ❖ Add all ingredients to a high speed blender and pulse until smooth.

Nutrition: Calories

Ingredients:
- ✓ 1 teaspoon of chia seeds
- ✓ 1½ cups of cold green tea
- ✓ ½ cup ice, crushed
- ❖ Pour the smoothie into two glasses and serve immediately.

91)   Cabbage and pineapple smoothie

Preparation time: 15 minutes   **Cooking time**:   **Servings**: 2

Ingredients:
- ✓ 1½ cups fresh cabbage, chopped and shredded
- ✓ 1 frozen banana, peeled and chopped
- ✓ ½ cup of fresh pineapple chunks

Directions:
- ❖ Add all ingredients to a high speed blender and pulse until smooth.

Nutrition: Calories

Ingredients:
- ✓ 1 cup unsweetened coconut milk
- ✓ ½ cup of fresh orange juice
- ✓ ½ cup of ice
- ❖ Pour the smoothie into two glasses and serve immediately.

92)   Green Vegetable Smoothie

Preparation time: 15 minutes   **Cooking time**:   **Servings**: 2

Ingredients:
- ✓ 1 medium avocado, peeled, pitted and chopped
- ✓ 1 large cucumber, peeled and chopped
- ✓ 2 fresh tomatoes, chopped
- ✓ 1 small green bell pepper, seeded and chopped

Directions:
- ❖ Add all ingredients to a high speed blender and pulse until smooth.

Nutrition: Calories

Ingredients:
- ✓ 1 cup fresh spinach, torn
- ✓ 2 tablespoons fresh lime juice
- ✓ 2 tablespoons of homemade vegetable broth
- ✓ 1 cup of alkaline water
- ❖ Pour smoothie into glasses and serve immediately.

93)   Avocado and spinach smoothie

Preparation time: 10 minutes   **Cooking time**:   **Servings**: 2

Ingredients:
- ✓ 2 cups of fresh spinach
- ✓ ½ avocado, peeled, pitted and chopped
- ✓ 4-6 drops of liquid stevia

Directions:
- ❖ Add all ingredients to a high speed blender and pulse until smooth.

Nutrition: Calories

Ingredients:
- ✓ ½ teaspoon ground cinnamon
- ✓ 1 tablespoon of hemp seeds
- ✓ 2 cups of cooled alkaline water
- ❖ Pour the smoothie into two glasses and serve immediately.

94)   Cucumber Smoothie

Preparation time: 15 minutes   **Cooking time**:   **Servings**: 2

Ingredients:
- ✓ 1 small cucumber, peeled and chopped
- ✓ 2 cups fresh mixed greens (spinach, kale, chard), chopped and shredded
- ✓ ½ cup of lettuce, torn
- ✓ ¼ cup fresh parsley leaves
- ✓ ¼ cup fresh mint leaves

Directions:
- ❖ Add all ingredients to a high speed blender and pulse until smooth.

Nutrition: Calories

Ingredients:
- ✓ 2-3 drops of liquid stevia
- ✓ 1 teaspoon fresh lemon juice
- ✓ 1½ cups of filtered water
- ✓ ¼ cup ice cubes

- ❖ Pour the smoothie into two glasses and serve immediately.

95)   Apple and Ginger Smoothie

Preparation time: 10 minutes   **Cooking time**: 0 minutes   **Servings**: 1

Ingredients:
- ✓ 1 apple, peeled and diced
- ✓ ¾ cup (6 ounces) of coconut yogurt

Directions:
- ❖ Add all ingredients to a blender.
- ❖ Blend well until smooth.

Nutrition: Calories

Ingredients:
- ✓ ½ teaspoon of ginger, freshly grated

- ❖ Refrigerate for 2 to 3 hours.
- ❖ Serve.

96)   Green Tea Blueberry Smoothie

Preparation time: 10 minutes   **Cooking time**: 5 minutes   **Servings**: 1

Ingredients:
- ✓ 3 tablespoons of alkaline water
- ✓ 1 green tea bag
- ✓ 1 ½ cups fresh blueberries

Directions:
- ❖ Boil 3 tablespoons of water in a small saucepan and transfer to a cup.
- ❖ Dip the tea bag into the cup and let it sit for 4 to 5 minutes.
- ❖ Discard the tea bag and
- ❖ Transfer the green tea to a blender

Nutrition: Calories

Ingredients:
- ✓ 1 pear, peeled, stoned and diced
- ✓ ¾ cup of almond milk

- ❖ Add all other ingredients to blender.
- ❖ Blend well until smooth.
- ❖ Serve with fresh blueberries.

97)　Apple and almond smoothie

Preparation time: 10 minutes   **Cooking time**: 0 minutes   **Servings: 1**

Ingredients:
- ✓ 1 cup of apple cider
- ✓ 1/2 cup of coconut yogurt
- ✓ 4 tablespoons almonds, crushed

Directions:
- ❖ Add all ingredients to a blender.

Nutrition: Calories

Ingredients:
- ✓ 1/4 teaspoon of cinnamon
- ✓ 1/4 teaspoon nutmeg
- ✓ 1 cup of ice cubes
- ❖ Blend well until smooth.
- ❖ Serve.

98)　Cranberry Smoothie

Preparation time: 10 minutes   **Cooking time**: 0 minutes   **Servings: 1**

Ingredients:
- ✓ 1 cup of cranberries
- ✓ ¾ cup of almond milk
- ✓ ¼ cup raspberries

Directions:
- ❖ Add all ingredients to a blender.

Nutrition: Calories

Ingredients:
- ✓ 2 teaspoons fresh ginger, finely grated
- ✓ 2 teaspoons of fresh lemon juice
- ❖ Blend well until smooth.
- ❖ Serve with fresh berries on top.

99)　Berry and Cinnamon Smoothie

Preparation time: 10 minutes   **Cooking time**: 0 minutes   **Servings: 1**

Ingredients:
- ✓ 1 cup of frozen strawberries
- ✓ 1 cup apple, peeled and diced
- ✓ 2 teaspoons fresh ginger
- ✓ 3 tablespoons of hemp seeds

Directions:
- ❖ Add all ingredients to a blender.

Nutrition: Calories

Ingredients:
- ✓ 1 cup of water
- ✓ ½ squeezed lime
- ✓ ¼ teaspoon of cinnamon powder
- ✓ ⅛ teaspoon of vanilla extract
- ❖ Blend well until smooth.
- ❖ Serve with fresh fruit

100)　Detoxifying Berry Smoothie

Preparation time: 10 minutes   **Cooking time**: 0 minutes   **Servings: 1**

Ingredients:
- ✓ 3 peaches, with stone and peel
- ✓ 5 blueberries

Directions:
- ❖ Add all ingredients to a blender.

Nutrition: Calories

Ingredients:
- ✓ 5 raspberries
- ✓ 1 cup of alkaline water
- ❖ Blend well until smooth.
- ❖ Serve with fresh kiwi wedges.

Chapter 7 - Dr. Lewis's Meal Plan Project

Day 1

1) Bowl Of Raspberry And Banana Smoothie

21) Tomato And Vegetable Salad

43) Spaghetti With Broccoli

62) Grilled Watermelon

85) Matcha Smoothie

Day 2

5) Spicy Quinoa Porridge

25) Curried Okra

48) Fresh Vegetarian Pizza

68) Dried Orange Slices

82) Kale Smoothie

Day 3

8) Fruity Oatmeal

28) Sauteed Mushrooms

56) Mint And Berry Soup

65) Roasted Chickpeas

94) Cucumber Smoothie

Day 4

11) Savory Sweet Potato Waffles

31) Roasted Butternut Squash

59) Mixed Mushroom Stew

74) Alka-Goulash Fast

91) Cabbage And Pineapple Smoothie

Day 5

14) Simple White Bread

34) Vegetarian Kebab

49) Spicy Lentil Burger

80) German Style Sweet Potato Salad

89) Mango Smoothie

Day 6

17) Granola With Coconut, Nuts And Seeds

37) Zoodles With Cream Sauce

57) Mushroom Soup

75) Eggplant Caviar

96) Green Tea Blueberry Smoothie

Day 7

20) Strawberry Sorbet

40) Vegetable Dish With Sesame

51) Sliced Sweet Potato With Artichoke Cream And Peppers

78) Hummus

99) Berry And Cinnamon Smoothie

Chapter 8 - Conclusion

I hope this book can lead you to your goals, keeping your desire to keep going high, without making you lose sight of the outcome

This book series is designed to help women, men, athletes and sportsmen, people immersed in work with little free time, etc.

If you recognize yourself in one of these categories or someone you know has decided to take the same path as you,

You'll find the other books in the series in your trusted bookstore, guaranteed!

Big hugs from Dr. Grace!

Alkaline Diet Cookbook for Men

Dr. Lewis's Meal Plan Project| 100 Specific Recipes to Keep Body Acids Under Control| Find the Well-Being You've Always Wished For Thanks to an Effective and Easy-To-Follow Path.

By Grace Lewis

Chapter 1 - Introduction

This book was written for all men who have made the choice to embark on a journey of transforming their lives.

The alkaline diet is the simplest and most effective way to begin a long-term journey of transformation.

Below we will answer some questions that people usually ask me during private sessions

What is an alkaline diet?

The premise of an alkaline diet is this: replace acidic foods with alkaline foods and your health will improve. Why would this work, you may ask? The theory is that by regulating your body's pH level (pH is a scientific scale on which acids and bases are measured), you can lose weight and avoid chronic diseases such as cancer and heart disease. pH is measured on a scale of 1 to 14; below seven are the most acidic foods, such as vinegar, animal fats and dairy products. Above seven are the alkaline foods, which mostly include healthy, plant-based foods. When we digest a food, we are left with residual ash, which can be acidic or alkaline. Therefore, an alkaline diet is sometimes called an alkaline ash diet. Proponents of the alkaline diet say that acidic ash can be dangerous to your health.

Is an alkaline diet healthy?

Processed meats are high on cancer doctors' list of foods never to eat, and they are also condemned in the alkaline diet because of their high acidity. "An alkaline diet is a diet that seeks to balance the body's pH levels by increasing the consumption of alkalizing foods such as fruits and vegetables and reducing/eliminating most acidifying foods such as processed meats and refined grains," explains Josh Axe, DNM, author of Eat Dirt and co-founder of Ancient Nutrition.

Can an alkaline diet reduce the risk of cancer?

Many anti-cancer foods are also alkaline diet foods, but there is currently no evidence for or against the role of alkaline diets in cancer prevention. However, plant-based diets are thought to help reduce the risk of cancer and are even recommended for cancer survivors, according to the American Institute for Cancer Research. New research from the University of Alabama at Birmingham suggests that a plant-based diet may make it easier to treat one of the deadliest forms of breast cancer. Although the evidence is somewhat contradictory: some chemotherapy drugs kill more cancer cells in an alkaline environment, while others work better in an acidic environment, according to a review in the Journal of Environmental Public Health. It's worth discussing this with your doctor if you are being treated for cancer.

At the end of the manual, you'll find my personal method designed for a male audience to get you started on the recipes in this book right away.

Enjoy!

Grace

Alkaline Diet Breakfast Recipes

1) Blueberry Muffins

Preparation time: 1 hour   **Cooking time**:   **Servings: 3**

Ingredients:
- ✓ 1/2 cup of Blueberries
- ✓ 3/4 cup of Teff Flour
- ✓ 3/4 cup of Spelt Flour
- ✓ 1/3 cup of Agave Syrup

Directions:
- ❖ Preheat our oven to 365 degrees Fahrenheit.
- ❖ Grate or line up 6 standard muffin cups.
- ❖ Add the yeast, sifted flour, sifted mashed potato, nut milk, peanut butter, and agave juice to a large bowl.

Nutrition: Calories

Helpful Hints:

Ingredients:
- ✓ 1/2 teaspoon of Pure Sea Salt
- ✓ 1 cup of Coconut Milk
- ✓ 1/4 cup Sea Moss Gel seed oil (optional, check information)

- ❖ Put them in order for a while.
- ❖ Add the blueberries to the mixture and mix well.
- ❖ Divide muffin batter among 6 muffin cups.
- ❖ Bake for 30 minutes until golden brown.
- ❖ Experiment and enjoy our Blueberry Muffins!

2) Banana Strawberry Ice Crem

Preparation time: **Cooking time**: 4 Hours   **Servings: 5**

Ingredients:
- ✓ 1 cup of Strawberry*.
- ✓ 5 quartered Baby Bananas*.
- ✓ 1/2 Avocado, chopped

Directions:
- ❖ Put all the ingredients in and let them dry well.
- ❖ Taste. If so, add more milk or agave syrup if you want it to be more full-bodied.

Nutrition: Calories

Ingredients:
- ✓ 1 tablespoon of Agave syrup
- ✓ 1/4 cup of walnut milk Homemade

- ❖ Place in a container with a lid and let mash for at least 5-6 hours.
- ❖ Serve and enjoy your Bana Strawberry Ice creamy!

Helpful hints: If you don't fresh berries or banas, you can use frozen ones. You can use as much fruit as you want, but be sure to use only fresh fruit. The fat in the Avocado helps make a creamier consisistency. If you don't have homemade nut milk, you can substitute it with homemade sheep's milk.

3) Chocolate cream Homemade Whipped

Preparation time: 10 Minutes.   **Cooking time**:   **Servings: 1 cup**

Ingredients:
- ✓ 1 cup of Aquafaba

Directions:
- ❖ Add Agave Syrup and Aquafaba into a bowl.
- ❖ Mix to the height speed about 5 minutes with a mixer stand o 10 to 15 minutes with a mixer hand.

Nutrition: Calories

Ingredients:
- ✓ 1/4 cup of Agave Syrup
- ❖ Serve and enjoy our Homemade Whipped Cream!

Helpful Hints: Keep in the refrigerator if not using immediately. The whipped cream will become Aquafaba consistency eventually, until set.

4) "Chocolate" Pudding.

Preparation time: **Cooking time:** 20 Minutes.   **Servings: 4**

Ingredients:
- ✓ 1 to 2 cups of Black Sapote
- ✓ 1/4 cup agave syrup
- ✓ 1/2 cup of soaked Brazil Nuts (overnight or at least 3 hours)

Directions:
- ❖ Cut 1 or 2 cups of Black Sapote in half.
- ❖ Remove all the seeds. You should have 1 cup ou full of fruit de-seded.

Nutrition: Calories

Ingredients:
- ✓ 1 tablespoon of hemp seeds
- ✓ 1/2 cup of Spring Water

- ❖ Place all ingredients in a blender and blend until smooth.
- ❖ Serve and enjoy our chocolate pudding!

Helpful Hints: Store in the refrigerator when not in use. You can use it with our Homemade whipped crust.

5) Walnut muffins

Preparation time: **Cooking time:** 1 hour   **Servings: 6**

Ingredients:
- ✓ Dry ingredients:
- ✓ 1 1/2 cups of Spell or Teff Flour
- ✓ 1/2 teaspoon of Pure Sea Salt
- ✓ 3/4 cup of Date Syrup
- ✓ What's the problem?
- ✓ 2 medium pureed Burro Banas

Directions:
- ❖ Preheat the oven to 400 degrees.
- ❖ Take a muffin tray and grease 12 cups or line with cupcake liners.
- ❖ Place all dry ingredients in a large bowl and mix well.
- ❖ Add all ingredients to a larger bowl and mix with the Bin Laden. 5. Mix the ingredients from the two bowls into one container. Be careful not to over mix.

Nutrition: Calories

Ingredients:
- ✓ ¼ cup of ground soybean oil
- ✓ ¾ cup of Homemade Walnut Milk *
- ✓ 1 tablespoon of Key Lime Juice
- ✓ Ingredients for filling:
- ✓ ½ cup of chopped Walnuts (plus extra for decorating)
- ✓ 1 banana burrita
- ❖ Add the filling ingredients and fry.
- ❖ Place our batter in the 12 muffin cups and fill them with a knob of butter.
- ❖ Bake 22 to 26 mnutes until golden brown.
- ❖ Allow to cool for 10 minutes.
- ❖ Serve and enjoy your Bana Nut Muffins!

Helpful Hints:

6) Banana and almond smoothie

Preparation time: 10 minutes   **Cooking time:** 0 minutes   **Servings: 2**

Ingredients:
- ✓ 2 large frozen bananas, peeled and sliced
- ✓ 1 tablespoon chopped almonds

Directions:
- ❖ Place all ingredients in a high speed blender and pulse until smooth and creamy.

Nutrition: Calories

Ingredients:
- ✓ 1 teaspoon of organic vanilla extract
- ✓ 2 cups of cooled unsweetened almond milk

- ❖ Pour smoothie into two serving glasses and serve immediately

7) Strawberry and Beet Smoothie

Preparation time: 10 minutes   **Cooking time:** 0 minutes   **Servings: 2**

Ingredients:
- ✓ 2 cups frozen strawberries, hulled
- ✓ 2/3 cup frozen beets, cut, peeled and chopped
- ✓ 1 teaspoon of fresh ginger root, peeled and grated

Directions:
- ❖ Place all ingredients in a high speed blender and pulse until smooth and creamy.

Nutrition: Calories

Ingredients:
- ✓ 1 teaspoon fresh turmeric root, peeled and grated
- ✓ ½ cup of fresh orange juice
- ✓ 1 cup unsweetened almond milk

- ❖ Pour smoothie into two serving glasses and serve immediately

8) Raspberry and tofu smoothie

Preparation time: 10 minutes   **Cooking time:**   **Servings: 2**

Ingredients:
- ✓ 1½ cups of fresh raspberries
- ✓ 6 ounces of firm silken tofu, drained, pressed and chopped
- ✓ 1 teaspoon of stevia powder

Directions:
- ❖ Place all ingredients in a high speed blender and pulse until smooth and creamy.

Nutrition: Calories

Ingredients:
- ✓ 1/8 teaspoon of organic vanilla extract
- ✓ 1½ cups unsweetened almond milk
- ✓ ¼ cup ice cubes, crushed

- ❖ Pour smoothie into two serving glasses and serve immediately

9) Mango and lemon smoothie

Preparation time: 10 minutes   **Cooking time:**   **Servings: 2**

Ingredients:
- ✓ 2 cups frozen mango, peeled, pitted and chopped
- ✓ ¼ cup almond butter
- ✓ pinch of ground turmeric

Directions:
- ❖ Place all ingredients in a high speed blender and pulse until smooth and creamy.

Nutrition: Calories

Ingredients:
- ✓ 2 tablespoons fresh lemon juice
- ✓ 1¼ cup unsweetened almond milk
- ✓ ¼ cup ice cubes, crushed

- ❖ Pour smoothie into two serving glasses and serve immediately

10)   Papaya and banana smoothie

Preparation time: 10 minutes   Cooking time: Servings: 2

Ingredients:
- ½ of a medium papaya, peeled and coarsely chopped
- 1 large banana, peeled and sliced
- 2 tablespoons of agave nectar
- ¼ teaspoon ground turmeric

Directions:
- Place all ingredients in a high speed blender and pulse until smooth and creamy.

Nutrition: Calories

Ingredients:
- 1 tablespoon fresh lime juice
- 1½ cups unsweetened almond milk
- ½ cup ice cubes, crushed

- Pour smoothie into two serving glasses and serve immediately

11)   Orange and Oat Smoothie

Preparation time: 10 minutes   Cooking time: Servings: 2

Ingredients:
- 2/3 cups rolled oats
- 2 oranges, peeled, with seeds and cut into pieces
- 2 large bananas, peeled and sliced

Directions:
- Place all ingredients in a high speed blender and pulse until smooth and creamy.

Nutrition: Calories

Ingredients:
- 1½ cups unsweetened almond milk
- ½ cup ice cubes, crushed

- Pour smoothie into two serving glasses and serve immediately

12)   Pineapple and Kale Smoothie

Preparation time: 10 minutes   Cooking time: Servings: 2

Ingredients:
- 1½ cups fresh cabbage, hard ribs removed and chopped
- 1 large frozen banana, peeled and sliced
- ½ cup fresh pineapple, peeled and cut into pieces

Directions:
- Place all ingredients in a high speed blender and pulse until smooth and creamy.

Nutrition: Calories

Ingredients:
- ½ cup of fresh orange juice
- 1 cup unsweetened coconut milk
- ½ cup ice cubes, crushed

- Pour smoothie into two serving glasses and serve immediately

13)   Pumpkin and Banana Smoothie

Preparation time: 10 minutes   Cooking time: Servings: 2

Ingredients:
- 1 cup homemade pumpkin puree
- 1 large banana, peeled and sliced
- 1 tablespoon maple syrup
- 1 teaspoon ground flax seeds

Directions:
- Place all ingredients in a high speed blender and pulse until smooth and creamy.

Nutrition: Calories

Ingredients:
- ¼ teaspoon of cinnamon powder
- 1/8 teaspoon ground ginger
- 1½ cups unsweetened almond milk
- ¼ cup ice cubes, crushed

- Pour smoothie into two serving glasses and serve immediately

14)   Cabbage and avocado smoothie

Preparation time: 10 minutes   **Cooking time**:   **Servings**: 2

Ingredients:
- ✓ 2 cups fresh cabbage, hard ribs removed and chopped
- ✓ ½ of a medium avocado, peeled, pitted and chopped
- ✓ ½ inch pieces of fresh ginger root, peeled and chopped

Directions:
- ❖ Place all ingredients in a high speed blender and pulse until smooth and creamy.

Nutrition: Calories

Ingredients:
- ✓ ½ inch pieces of fresh turmeric root, peeled and chopped
- ✓ 1½ cups unsweetened coconut milk
- ✓ ¼ cup ice cubes, crushed
- ❖ Pour smoothie into two serving glasses and serve immediately

15)   Cucumber and Herb Smoothie

Preparation time: 10 minutes   **Cooking time**:   **Servings**: 2

Ingredients:
- ✓ 2 cups fresh mixed vegetables (cabbage, beets), chopped and shredded
- ✓ 1 small cucumber, peeled and chopped
- ✓ ½ cup of lettuce, torn
- ✓ ¼ cup fresh parsley leaves
- ✓ ¼ cup fresh mint leaves

Directions:
- ❖ Place all ingredients in a high speed blender and pulse until smooth and creamy.

Nutrition: Calories

Ingredients:
- ✓ 2-3 drops of liquid stevia
- ✓ 1 teaspoon fresh lemon juice
- ✓ 1½ cups of alkaline water
- ✓ ¼ cup ice cubes, crushed

16)   Hemp seed and carrot muffins

Pour smoothie into two serving glasses and serve immediately

Preparation time: 20-25 minutes   **Cooking time**:   **Servings**: 12

Ingredients:
- ✓ Cashew butter, 6 tablespoons
- ✓ Shredded Carrot,
- ✓ Unrefined whole cane sugar, .5 c.
- ✓ Almond milk, 1 c.
- ✓ Oatmeal, 2 c.
- ✓ Ground flaxseed, 1 tablespoon

Directions:
- ❖ Start by setting your oven to 350.
- ❖ Whisk the flax seeds and water together to make the flax egg.
- ❖ Pour everything into a larger bowl and then combine the salt, vanilla powder, baking powder, kale, hemp seeds, cashew butter, carrot, sugar, almond milk and oatmeal.

Nutrition: Calories

Ingredients:
- ✓ Water, 3 tablespoons
- ✓ Pinch of sea salt
- ✓ Powdered vanilla bean, one pinch
- ✓ Baking powder, 1 tablespoon
- ✓ Chopped cabbage, 1 tablespoon
- ✓ Hemp seeds, 2 tablespoons
- ❖ Mix everything together until well combined.
- ❖ Grease a 12-cup muffin pan and divide the batter between the cups. Bake for 20-25 minutes and enjoy.

17)   Chia seed and strawberry parfait

Preparation time:	Cooking time:	Servings: 2

Ingredients:
- ✓ Strawberry mixture -
- ✓ Brown rice syrup, 1-2 teaspoons
- ✓ Chia seeds, 1 teaspoon
- ✓ Diced strawberries, 1 c.
- ✓ Oat Blend -

Directions:
- ❖ To make the strawberry mixture, mix together the brown rice syrup, chia seeds and strawberries in a small bowl until well blended.
- ❖ In a separate bowl, mix together the vanilla bean powder, brown rice syrup, coconut milk and oats until well blended.

Nutrition: Calories

Ingredients:
- ✓ Quick rolled oats, 1 c.
- ✓ Powdered vanilla bean, one pinch
- ✓ Brown rice syrup, 1 tablespoon
- ✓ Coconut milk, 1 c.

- ❖ Place one part of the oats in the base of two jars. Cover with some of the strawberry mixture. Repeat with the remaining ingredients.
- ❖ Put a lid on the jars and let them sit in the fridge overnight.
- ❖ The next morning, discover and enjoy.

18)   Pecan Pancakes

Preparation time:	Cooking time:	Servings: 5

Ingredients:
- ✓ Chopped pecans, .25 c.
- ✓ Nutmeg, .25 tsp
- ✓ Cinnamon, 0.5 teaspoons
- ✓ Vanilla, 1 teaspoon
- ✓ Melted butter, 2 tablespoons
- ✓ Unsweetened soy milk, .75 c.

Directions:
- ❖ Place the salt, sugar substitute, baking powder and almond flour in a bowl and mix well.
- ❖ In another bowl, place the vanilla, soy milk, butter and eggs. Stir well to incorporate everything.
- ❖ Place the egg mixture into the dry contents and mix well until well blended.
- ❖ Add the nutmeg, pecans and cinnamon. Stir for five minutes.

Ingredients:
- ✓ Eggs, 2
- ✓ Salt, .25 tsp
- ✓ Baking powder, .25 tsp
- ✓ Granular sugar substitute, 1 tablespoon
- ✓ Almond flour, .75 c.
- ✓ Olive oil - cooking spray

- ❖ Place a 12-inch skillet over medium heat and sprinkle with cooking spray.
- ❖ Pour one tablespoon of batter into the preheated pan and spread into a four-inch circle.
- ❖ Pour three more spoonfuls into the pan and cook until bubbles have formed at the edges of the pancakes and the bottom is golden brown.
- ❖ Turn each one over and cook an additional two minutes.
- ❖ Repeat the process until all the batter has been used.
- ❖ Serve with a syrup of your choice.

Nutrition: Calories

19)   Quinoa Breakfast

Preparation time:	Cooking time:	Servings: 4

Ingredients:
- ✓ Maple syrup, 3 tablespoons
- ✓ 2 inch cinnamon stick
- ✓ Water, 2 c.
- ✓ Quinoa, 1 c.
- ✓ Optional Condiments:
- ✓ Yogurt
- ✓ Chopped cashews, 2 tablespoons

Directions:
- ❖ Place the quinoa in a colander and rinse under cold running water. Make sure there are no stones or anything else.
- ❖ Pour the water into a saucepan, add the quinoa and place the saucepan over medium heat. Bring to a boil.

Nutrition: Calories

Ingredients:
- ✓ Whipped coconut cream, 3 tablespoons
- ✓ Lime juice, 1 teaspoon
- ✓ Nutmeg, .25 tsp
- ✓ Raisins, 2 tablespoons
- ✓ Strawberries, .5 c.
- ✓ Raspberries, .5 c.
- ✓ Blueberries, .5 c.
- ❖ Add the cinnamon stick, put a lid on the saucepan, lower the hot temperature, even, simmer gently fifteen minutes until the water is engulfed.
- ❖ Remove from hot temperature and stir with a fork. Add maple syrup and one of the toppings listed above.

20)   Oatmeal

Preparation time: **Cooking time**:   **Servings: 4**

Ingredients:
- ✓ Halls
- ✓ Steel cut oats, 1.25 c.
- ✓ Water, 3.75 c.
- ✓ Optional Condiments:
- ✓ Nuts
- ✓ Dried fruits
- ✓ Sliced banana
- ✓ Mango cubes

Ingredients:
- ✓ Mixed berries
- ✓ Garam masala, 1 teaspoon
- ✓ Lemon pepper, .25 tsp
- ✓ Nutmeg, .25 tsp
- ✓ Cinnamon, 1 teaspoon

Directions:
- ❖ Place a saucepan on medium and add the water. Allow the water to boil.
- ❖ Pour in the oats with a pinch of salt and lower the heat to a simmer.

- ❖ Let simmer 25 minutes, stirring constantly.
- ❖ Once all the water has been absorbed, add one of the seasonings listed above if you want to add some flavor. If you want it creamier, add a tablespoon of coconut milk.

Nutrition: Calories

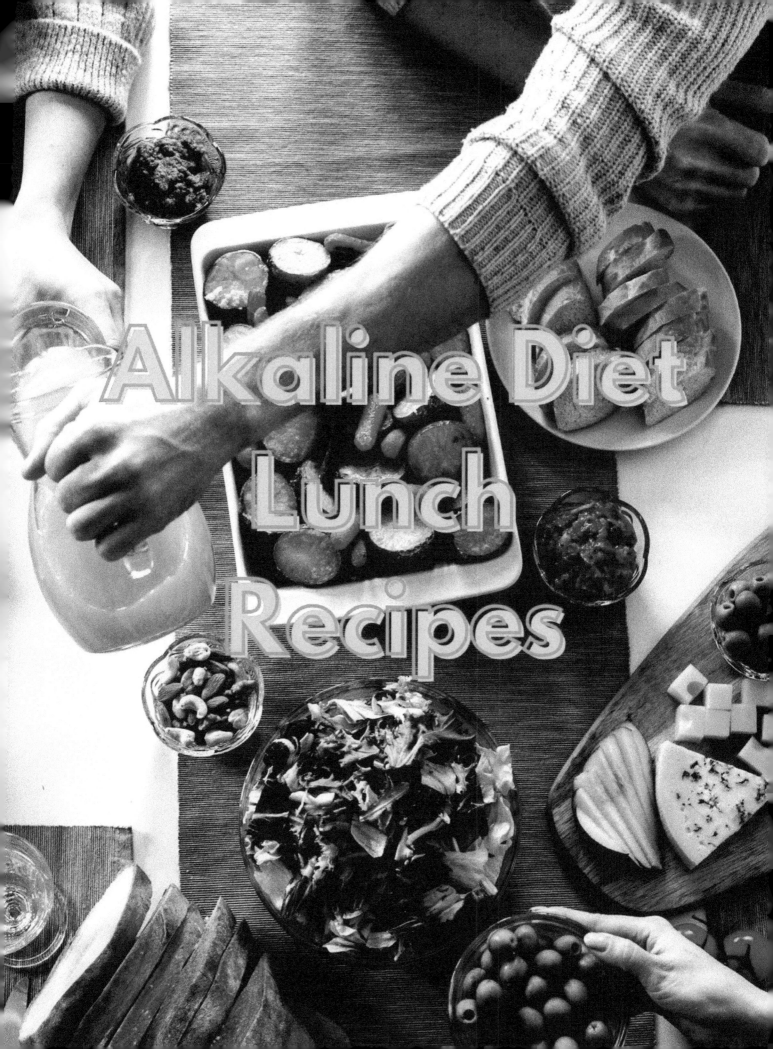

21)   Sweet spinach salad

Preparation time: **Cooking time:**   **Portions:**

Ingredients:
- ✓ Crushed black pepper (1 teaspoon)
- ✓ Salt (1 teaspoon)
- ✓ Nutmeg (1 teaspoon)
- ✓ Cinnamon (1 teaspoon)
- ✓ Chopped spinach (4 c.)
- ✓ Chopped parsley (2 tablespoons)

Directions:
- ❖ To start this recipe, bring out a large bowl and combine all the ingredients together.

Nutrition: Calories

Ingredients:
- ✓ Chopped walnuts (.25 c.)
- ✓ Raisins (.25 c.)
- ✓ Sliced apple (.5 c.)
- ✓ Yogurt (.5 c.)
- ✓ Lime juice (1 tablespoon)
- ✓ Shredded carrots (.75 c.)
- ❖ Place the bowl in the refrigerator to chill for about ten minutes before serving.

22)   Steamed green bowl

Preparation time: **Cooking time:**   **Portions:**

Ingredients:
- ✓ Chopped coriander (2 tablespoons)
- ✓ Salt (1 teaspoon)
- ✓ Sliced green onions (2)
- ✓ Ground cashews (1 c.)
- ✓ Coconut milk (2 c.)
- ✓ Green peas (.5 c.)
- ✓ Sliced zucchini (1)

Directions:
- ❖ Heat some coconut oil in a pan and when hot, add the ginger, turmeric, garlic and onion.
- ❖ After five minutes of cooking, add the coconut milk, peas, zucchini and broccoli to this mixture.

Nutrition: Calories

Ingredients:
- ✓ Head of broccoli (1)
- ✓ Grated ginger (1 inch)
- ✓ Turmeric (1 teaspoon)
- ✓ Chopped garlic clove (1)
- ✓ Sliced onion (1)
- ✓ Coconut oil (1 tablespoon)

- ❖ Let the ingredients come to a boil before reducing the heat and simmering for a bit.
- ❖ After another 15 minutes, stir in the cilantro, salt, green onions and cashews before serving.

23)   Vegetable and berry salad

Preparation time: **Cooking time:**   **Portions:**

Ingredients:
- ✓ Raspberries (.5 c.)
- ✓ Sliced tangerine (.5)
- ✓ Alfalfa sprouts (1 c.)
- ✓ Shredded red cabbage (.5 head)
- ✓ Lemon juice 1)
- ✓ Olive oil (3 tablespoons)
- ✓ Diced cucumber (1)
- ✓ Avocado (1)
- ✓ Sliced shallot (1)

Directions:
- ❖ Take a large bowl and add all the ingredients to it.

Nutrition: Calories

Ingredients:
- ✓ Sliced cabbage (4 leaves)
- ✓ Chopped parsley (1 tablespoon)
- ✓ Sliced red bell pepper (.5)
- ✓ Shredded Carrot (1)
- ✓ Crushed almonds (1 tablespoon)
- ✓ Pumpkin seeds (2 tablespoons)

- ❖ Stir well to combine before seasoning the fruits and vegetables with a little lemon juice and a little oil.
- ❖ Serve immediately.

24)   Bowl of quinoa and carrots

Preparation time: **Cooking time**:   **Portions**:

Ingredients:
- ✓ Sliced green onions (2 tablespoons)
- ✓ Black sesame seeds (2 tablespoons)
- ✓ Salt (.25 tsp.)
- ✓ Chopped parsley (3 tablespoons)
- ✓ Lemon juice (.5)
- ✓ Cooked quinoa (2 c.)

Directions:
- ❖ Whisk together the miso and water in a bowl. Then take a frying pan and heat some oil in it.
- ❖ When the oil is hot, add the fennel bulb and carrots and cook for a few minutes, turning when three minutes have passed.

Ingredients:
- ✓ Sliced fennel bulb (1)
- ✓ Carrots, chopped (1 bunch)
- ✓ Olive oil (1 tablespoon)
- ✓ Miso (1 tablespoon)
- ✓ Water (1 c.)

- ❖ Add the water and miso mixture to the pan and reduce the heat to low. Cook with the lid on for a bit. This will take about 20 minutes.
- ❖ While this mixture is cooking, combine together the quinoa with the parsley, lemon juice and salt in a bowl.
- ❖ When the carrots are done, add the mixture on top of the quinoa. Sprinkle the green onions and sesame seeds on top before serving.

Nutrition: Calories

25)   Grab and Go Wraps

Preparation time: **Cooking time**:   **Portions**:

Ingredients:
- ✓ Carrot cut into julienne (1)
- ✓ Red bell pepper (.5)
- ✓ Swiss chard greens (4)
- ✓ Salt (.25 tsp.)
- ✓ Diced jalapeno bell pepper (.5)

Directions:
- ❖ Get out your blender or food processor and combine together the salt, jalapeno, shallots, cilantro, lime, avocado and peas. Process to combine, but leave some texture to still be there.

Ingredients:
- ✓ Shallots cut into small cubes (1)
- ✓ Chopped coriander leaves (.25 c.)
- ✓ Lime Juice (1)
- ✓ Avocado (1)
- ✓ Steamed green peas (1 c.)
- ❖ Lay the collards out on the counter and then spread your pea and avocado mixture on top.
- ❖ Add the carrot and bell bell pepper strips before rolling up the collars and secure with a toothpick.
- ❖ Repeat with all ingredients before serving.

Nutrition: Calories

26)   Walnut Tacos

Preparation time: **Cooking time**:   **Portions**:

Ingredients:
- ✓ Chopped coriander (1 tablespoon)
- ✓ Nutritional yeast (2 tablespoons)
- ✓ Romaine lettuce leaves (6)
- ✓ Cooked red quinoa (.25 c.)
- ✓ Salt (.25 tsp.)
- ✓ Tamari (1 tablespoon)
- ✓ Coconut amino acids (1 teaspoon)
- ✓ Smoked paprika (.25 tsp.)

Directions:
- ❖ To start this recipe, add the almonds and walnuts to the food processor and puree them.
- ❖ Add the tomatoes and give it a couple of pulses until you have a nice crumbly mixture.
- ❖ From there, add the salt, tamari, coconut aminos, paprika, onion, garlic, chili, cilantro, cumin, and olive oil.

Nutrition: Calories

Ingredients:
- ✓ Onion powder (.25 tsp.)
- ✓ Garlic Powder (.25 tsp.)
- ✓ Chilli powder (.25 tsp.)
- ✓ Ground Coriander (1 teaspoon)
- ✓ Ground Cumin (1 teaspoon)
- ✓ Olive oil (2 tablespoons)
- ✓ Chopped dried tomatoes (.25 c.)
- ✓ Chopped raw almonds (.25 c.)
- ✓ Walnuts (.5 c.)
- ❖ It pulses a few more times to be fully combined.
- ❖ Add the tomato and walnut mixture to a bowl and combine with the quinoa.
- ❖ Divide this mixture among the romaine lettuce leaves and top with the cilantro and nutritional yeast before serving.

27)   Tex-Mex bowl

Preparation time: **Cooking time:**   **Portions:**

Ingredients:
- ✓ Nutritional yeast (2 tablespoons)
- ✓ Cilantro (2 tablespoons)
- ✓ Sliced avocado (1)
- ✓ Salt (.25 tsp.)
- ✓ Olive oil (.25 c.)
- ✓ Apple Cider Vinegar (.25 c.)
- ✓ Lime juice and zest (1)
- ✓ Lemon juice and zest (1)
- ✓ Squeezed Oranges (2)
- ✓ Chopped garlic cloves (2)
- ✓ Sliced red onion (1)
- ✓ Sliced peppers
- ✓ For the brown rice
- ✓ Hind beans (.5 c.)

Ingredients:
- ✓ Garlic powder (.5 tsp.)
- ✓ Cayenne pepper (.5 tsp.)
- ✓ Paprika (1 teaspoon)
- ✓ Salt (1 teaspoon)
- ✓ Garlic powder (1.5 teaspoons)
- ✓ Chili powder (2 teaspoons)
- ✓ Cooked brown rice (1 c.)
- ✓ Sauce
- ✓ Juice of a lime
- ✓ Salt (.25 tsp.)
- ✓ Diced Cilantro (.25 c.)
- ✓ Diced red onion (.5)
- ✓ Diced Tomatoes (2)

Directions:
- ❖ Pull out a large bowl and combine together the salt, olive oil, vinegar, lime zest and juice, lemon zest and juice, garlic, red onion, and bell bell pepper.
- ❖ Cover and let sit for about five hours to marinate a bit. While the peppers marinate a bit in the refrigerator, it's time to work on the sauce.
- ❖ To make the sauce, add all ingredients to a small bowl and mix well to combine. Cover the bowl and place in the refrigerator.

- ❖ In a medium bowl, add all the ingredients for the brown rice. Mix well and set aside.
- ❖ Heat your skillet and add the peppers with some of the marinade. Cook for a bit until the onion and peppers are soft.
- ❖ Add the rice to a few serving bowls and top with the bell pepper and onion mixture, salsa and avocado. Add the nutritional yeast and cilantro before serving.

Nutrition: Calories

28)   Avocado and salmon soup

Preparation time: **Cooking time:**   **Portions:**

Ingredients:
- ✓ Cilantro (2 tablespoons)
- ✓ Crushed pepper (1 teaspoon)
- ✓ Olive oil (1 tablespoon)
- ✓ Flaked salmon (1 can)
- ✓ Salt (.25 tsp.)
- ✓ Cumin (.25 tsp.)
- ✓ Vegetable stock (1.5 c.)

Ingredients:
- ✓ Whole coconut cream (2 tablespoons)
- ✓ Lemon juice (4 tablespoons)
- ✓ Sliced green onion (1 tablespoon)
- ✓ Chopped Shallot (1)
- ✓ Pitted Avocado (3)

Directions:
- ❖ Take out a blender and combine together the salt, cumin, vegetable broth, coconut cream, two tablespoons of lemon juice, green onion, scallion, and avocado.
- ❖ Blend until smooth and then chill in the refrigerator for an hour.

- ❖ Meanwhile, take a bowl and combine together a tablespoon of cilantro, two tablespoons of lemon juice, the pepper, olive oil and salmon.
- ❖ Add the cooled avocado soup to the bowls and top each with the salmon and the rest of the cilantro. Serve immediately.

Nutrition: Calories

29)   Asian Pumpkin Salad

Preparation time: **Cooking time:**   **Portions:**

Ingredients:
- ✓ Diced avocado (.5)
- ✓ Pomegranate seeds (.25 c.)
- ✓ Lemon juice (1 tablespoon)
- ✓ Sliced cabbage (4 c.)
- ✓ Olive oil (1.5 tablespoons)
- ✓ Diced pumpkin (2 c.)
- ✓ Salt (.5 tsp.)

Ingredients:
- ✓ Red pepper flakes (.25 tsp.)
- ✓ Ground mustard (.25 tsp.)
- ✓ Ground Garlic (.25 tsp.)
- ✓ Ground cloves (.25 tsp.)
- ✓ Black sesame seeds (1 tablespoon)
- ✓ White sesame seeds (1 tablespoon)

Directions:
- ❖ Turn on the oven and give it time to heat to 400 degrees. Prepare a baking sheet with baking paper.
- ❖ In a large dish, combine the black and white sesame seeds with the salt, chili flakes, mustard, garlic and cloves.
- ❖ Drizzle the squash with a little olive oil and then roll each cube in the sesame seed mixture, pressing down a little to coat it.

- ❖ Add the squash to the baking dish and place it in the oven. It will take about half an hour to bake.
- ❖ While the squash is cooking, add the kale to a large bowl and pour in the salt, lemon juice and the rest of the olive oil. Massage the mixture into the kale and then set aside.
- ❖ When the squash is ready, add it on top of the kale and garnish with the avocado and pomegranate seeds before serving.

Nutrition: Calories

30)   Sweet potato rolls

Preparation time: **Cooking time:**   **Portions:**

Ingredients:
- ✓ Avocado (1)
- ✓ Alfalfa sprouts (1 c.)
- ✓ Sliced red onion (.5)
- ✓ Spinach (1 c.)
- ✓ Cooked quinoa (.5 c.)
- ✓ Swiss chard greens (4)
- ✓ Sweet potato hummus
- ✓ Crushed black pepper (.25 tsp.)

Ingredients:
- ✓ Salt (.25 tsp.)
- ✓ Cinnamon powder (.25 tsp.)
- ✓ Chilli powder (.25 tsp.)
- ✓ Garlic clove (1)
- ✓ Lemon juice (.5)
- ✓ Olive oil (.25 c.)
- ✓ Tahini (.33 c.)
- ✓ Diced sweet potato (1)
- ❖ Process until the mixture is smooth.
- ❖ Lay out each of the green collars and then spread sweet potato hummus on each.
- ❖ Add the avocado, sprouts, onion, spinach and quinoa. Roll everything up and secure with toothpicks. Repeat until the vegetables and filling are done.

Directions:
- ❖ Take the sweet potatoes and add them to a pan. Cover with water and bring to a boil. When it reaches a boil, reduce the flame and let it cook for a while to make the potatoes tender.
- ❖ When these are ready, drain the water and add them to the food processor along with pepper, salt, cinnamon, chili powder, garlic, lemon juice, olive oil and tahini.

Nutrition: Calories

31)   Spicy cabbage bowl

Preparation time: **Cooking time:**   **Portions:**

Ingredients:
- ✓ Sesame seeds (1 tablespoon)
- ✓ Green onion (.25 c.)
- ✓ Cabbage (2 c.)
- ✓ Coconut amino acids (1 teaspoon)
- ✓ Tamari (2 tablespoons)
- ✓ Chopped kimchi cabbage (1 c.)

Ingredients:
- ✓ Cooked brown rice (1 c.)
- ✓ Chopped garlic (1 teaspoon)
- ✓ Grated ginger (.5 tsp.)
- ✓ Sesame oil (2 tablespoons)

Directions:
- ❖ Take out a frying pan and heat the sesame oil in it. When the oil is hot, add together the coconut amino acid, tamari, kimchi, brown rice, garlic and ginger.

- ❖ After five minutes of cooking these ingredients, add the green onions and cabbage and toss to combine.
- ❖ Cook for a little longer. Then you can garnish the dish with some sesame seeds before serving.

Nutrition: Calories

32)   Citrus and fennel salad

Preparation time: **Cooking time:**   **Portions:**

Ingredients:
- ✓ Diced avocado (.5)
- ✓ Pomegranate seeds (2 tablespoons)
- ✓ Pepper (.5 tsp.)
- ✓ Salt (.25 tsp.)
- ✓ Olive oil (.25 c.)
- ✓ Orange juice (2 tablespoons)
- ✓ Lemon juice (2 tablespoons)

Directions:
- ❖ To start this recipe, bring out a large bowl and combine together the parsley, mint, fennel slices, grapefruit wedges, and orange wedges. Stir to combine.
- ❖ In another bowl, whisk together the pepper, salt, olive oil, orange juice and lemon juice.

Nutrition: Calories

Ingredients:
- ✓ Chopped mint (1 tablespoon)
- ✓ Chopped parsley (.5 c.)
- ✓ Sliced fennel bulbs (2)
- ✓ Red grapefruit segmented (.5)
- ✓ Segmented orange (1)

- ❖ Once combined, pour over the fennel and citrus mixture in the large bowl, stirring to coat.
- ❖ Move to a plate and garnish with the avocado and pomegranate seeds. Serve immediately.

33)   Vegan Burger

Preparation time: **Cooking time:**   **Servings: 4 hamburger patties**

Ingredients:
- ✓ 1/4 to 1/2 cup of spring water
- ✓ 1/2 teaspoon of cayenne powder
- ✓ 1/2 teaspoon of ginger powder
- ✓ Grape oil
- ✓ 1 teaspoon of dill
- ✓ 2 teaspoons of sea salt
- ✓ 2 teaspoons of onion powder

Directions:
- ❖ Mix the vegetables and seasonings in a large bowl, then add the flour. Gently add the spring water and stir the mixture until combined. If the mixture is too soft, add more flour.

Nutrition: Calories

Ingredients:
- ✓ 2 teaspoons of oregano
- ✓ 2 teaspoons of basil
- ✓ ¼ cup cherry tomatoes, diced
- ✓ 1/2 cup of cabbage, diced
- ✓ 1/2 cup green peppers, diced
- ✓ 1/2 cup onions, diced
- ✓ 1 cup of chickpea flour

- ❖ Divide the dough into 4 meatballs. Cook patties in grapeseed oil, in a skillet over medium heat for about 2 to 3 minutes per side. Continue flipping until the burger is brown on all sides.
- ❖ Serve the burger on a bun and enjoy.

34)   Alkaline spicy cabbage

Preparation time: **Cooking time:**   **Servings: 1 portion**

Ingredients:
- ✓ Grape oil
- ✓ 1/4 teaspoon of sea salt
- ✓ 1 teaspoon crushed red pepper

Directions:
- ❖ First wash the cabbage well and then fold each cabbage leaf in half. Cut off and discard the stems. Cut the prepared cabbage into bite-size portions and use the salad spinner to remove the water.
- ❖ In a wok, add 2 tablespoons of grapeseed oil and heat the oil over high heat.

Nutrition: Calories

Ingredients:
- ✓ 1/4 cup red bell bell pepper, diced
- ✓ 1/4 cup onion, diced
- ✓ 1 bunch of cabbage

- ❖ Fry the peppers and onions in the oil for about 2-3 minutes and then season with a little sea salt.
- ❖ Lower the heat and add the cabbage, cover the wok with a lid and simmer for about 5 minutes.
- ❖ Open the lid and add the crushed pepper, mix well and cover again. Cook until tender, or about 3 more minutes.

35) Electric Salad

Preparation time: **Cooking time:**   **Servings: 4**

Ingredients:
- ✓ 3 jalapenos
- ✓ 2 red onions
- ✓ 1 orange bell pepper
- ✓ 1 yellow bell pepper
- ✓ 1 cup cherry tomatoes, chopped

Directions:
- ❖ First wash and rinse the ingredients well. Dry the ingredients and then cut them into bite-size pieces, or as required.

Nutrition: Calories

Ingredients:
- ✓ 1 bunch of cabbage
- ✓ 1 handful of romaine lettuce
- ✓ Extra virgin olive oil
- ✓ Juice of 1 lime

- ❖ Place ingredients in a bowl and drizzle with olive oil and lime juice to your preferred taste.

36) Kale salad

Preparation time: **Cooking time:**   **Servings: 2**

Ingredients:
- ✓ 1/4 teaspoon of cayenne
- ✓ 1/2 teaspoon of sea salt
- ✓ 1/2 cup of cooked chickpeas
- ✓ 1/2 cup of red onions
- ✓ 1/2 cup sliced red, orange, yellow and green peppers
- ✓ 4 cups chopped cabbage

Directions:
- ❖ In a bowl, mix all the ingredients for the coleslaw and toss.

Nutrition: Calories

Ingredients:
- ✓ 1/2 cup alkaline garlic sauce (recipe included).
- ✓ Alkaline Garlic Sauce
- ✓ 1/4 teaspoon of dill
- ✓ 1/4 teaspoon of sea salt
- ✓ 1/2 teaspoon of ginger
- ✓ 1 tablespoon of onion powder
- ✓ 1/4 cup shallots, chopped
- ✓ 1 cup of grape oil
- ❖ Prepare the dressing by mixing the ingredients for the "Alkaline Electric Garlic Sauce".
- ❖ Drizzle with half a cup of sauce and then serve.

37) Walnut, date, orange and cabbage salad

Preparation time: **Cooking time:**   **Servings: 2**

Ingredients:
- ✓ /2 red onion, very thinly sliced
- ✓ 2 bunches of cabbage, or 6 full cups of sprouts
- ✓ 6 medjool dates, pitted
- ✓ 1/3 cup whole walnuts
- ✓ For the dressing

Directions:
- ❖ Preheat the oven to 375 degrees F and then place the walnuts on a baking sheet. Roast the walnuts for about 7-8 minutes, or until the skin begins to darken and crack.
- ❖ Once done, transfer the walnuts while still warm and let them steam for 15 minutes wrapped in a kitchen towel.
- ❖ Once cooled, squeeze and turn firmly to remove the skin, all still wrapped in the towel.
- ❖ In a food processor, place the pitted dates along with the walnuts and puree until fully blended and finely chopped. Set aside to cover the salad.

Nutrition: Calories

Ingredients:
- ✓ 5 tablespoons of olive oil
- ✓ Pinch of coarse salt
- ✓ 1 medjool date
- ✓ 4 tablespoons of freshly squeezed orange juice
- ✓ 2 tablespoons of lime juice
- ❖ Then wash, dry and cut the cabbage and place in a large bowl. Thinly slice the onion and add it to the bowl.
- ❖ Now prepare the dressing by combining the ingredients for the "dressing" in the blender apart from the olive oil.
- ❖ Blend the mixture to break up the dates and then pour in the oil in a steady stream to emulsify the dressing.
- ❖ Finally, toss the cabbage and onion mixture with the orange and walnut dressing.
- ❖ Move to a serving bowl and sprinkle with the walnut and date mixture. Enjoy!

38) Tomatoes with basil-snack

Preparation time:	Cooking time:	Servings: 1 portion

Ingredients:
- ✓ ¼ teaspoon of sea salt
- ✓ 2 tablespoons of lemon juice
- ✓ 2 tablespoons of olive oil

Directions:
- ❖ Start by slicing the cherry tomatoes and placing them in a medium sized bowl.
- ❖ Then finely chop your basil and add it to the bowl of tomatoes.

Nutrition: Calories

Ingredients:
- ✓ ¼ cup basil, fresh
- ✓ 1 cup chopped tomatoes, cherry or Roma

- ❖ Drizzle the tomatoes and basil with a little olive oil and lemon juice.
- ❖ Add a little sea salt to taste.
- ❖ Serve.

39) Pasta with spelt, zucchini and eggplant

Preparation time:	Cooking time:	Servings: 4

Ingredients:
- ✓ 2 teaspoons of dried basil leaves
- ✓ 1 teaspoon of oregano
- ✓ 2/3 cup vegetable broth
- ✓ 2/3 cup of dried and diced cherry tomatoes
- ✓ 1 large zucchini, diced
- ✓ 3 medium-sized, ripe cherry tomatoes, diced

Directions:
- ❖ Over medium heat, heat a little oil in a skillet and then sauté the eggplant, ginger and onion for about 8-10 minutes, stirring constantly.
- ❖ Then add the oregano, tomatoes and zucchini and let cook for 6-8 minutes, stirring occasionally.

Nutrition: Calories

Ingredients:
- ✓ 2-3 ginger, crushed
- ✓ 1-2 white onions, finely chopped
- ✓ 3 tablespoons of cold-pressed extra virgin olive oil
- ✓ 1 large eggplant cut into cubes
- ✓ 300g of spelt pasta
- ✓ Sea salt to taste
- ❖ Now heat the water and cook the pasta until it is firm to the bite, and then add the vegetable broth to the pan.
- ❖ Season with fresh pepper, salt and dried basil. Allow the mixture to simmer for a few minutes, covered.
- ❖ Once cooked, you can serve the sauce over pasta and garnish with fresh basil leaves.

40) Alkalizing millet dish

Preparation time:	Cooking time:	Servings: 2

Ingredients:
- ✓ 1/2 teaspoon of sea salt
- ✓ 2 1/2 cups of water

Directions:
- ❖ In a pot with an airtight lid, add the millet and then sauté over medium heat, stirring constantly.
- ❖ As soon as the millet turns golden brown, add the sea salt and water and cover the ingredients with a lid.
- ❖ Then bring the mixture to a boil and let it simmer until all the water has been absorbed, or for about 25-35 minutes.

Nutrition: Calories

Ingredients:
- ✓ 1 cup millet

- ❖ Alternatively, you can cook on an electric stove. Just cover the lid and bring to a boil, simmer for a couple of minutes and then turn off the stove.
- ❖ Allow the contents to cool for about 30 minutes with the lid on to allow the millet to dry out.
- ❖ Then serve and enjoy the millet.

Alkaline Diet Dinner Recipes

41)   Mixed stew of spicy vegetables

Preparation time: 20 minutes   **Cooking time**: 35 minutes   **Servings**: 8

Ingredients:
- ✓ 2 tablespoons of coconut oil
- ✓ 1 large sweet onion, chopped
- ✓ 1 medium parsnip, peeled and chopped
- ✓ 3 tablespoons of homemade tomato paste
- ✓ 2 large garlic cloves, minced
- ✓ ½ teaspoon of cinnamon powder
- ✓ ½ teaspoon ground ginger
- ✓ 1 teaspoon of ground cumin
- ✓ ¼ teaspoon cayenne pepper

Directions:
- ❖ In a large soup pot, melt the coconut oil over medium-high heat and sauté the onion for about 5 minutes.
- ❖ Add the parsnips and sauté for about 3 minutes.
- ❖ Add the tomato paste, garlic and spices and sauté for 2 minutes.

Ingredients:
- ✓ 2 medium carrots, peeled and chopped
- ✓ 2 medium purple potatoes, peeled and cut into pieces
- ✓ 2 medium sweet potatoes, peeled and cut into pieces
- ✓ 4 cups of homemade vegetable broth
- ✓ 2 tablespoons fresh lemon juice
- ✓ 2 cups fresh cabbage, hard ribs removed and chopped
- ✓ ¼ cup fresh parsley leaves, chopped

- ❖ Stir in the carrots, potatoes, sweet potatoes and broth and bring to a boil.
- ❖ Reduce heat to medium-low and simmer, covered for about 20 minutes.
- ❖ Add the lemon juice and cabbage and simmer for 5 minutes.
- ❖ Serve with a garnish of parsley.

Nutrition: Calories

42)   Mixed vegetable stew with herbs

Preparation time: 15 minutes   **Cooking time**: 2¼ hours   **Servings**: 8

Ingredients:
- ✓ 2 tablespoons of coconut oil
- ✓ 1 medium yellow onion, chopped
- ✓ 2 cups celery, chopped
- ✓ ½ teaspoon of minced garlic
- ✓ 3 cups fresh cabbage, hard ribs removed and chopped
- ✓ ½ cup fresh mushrooms, sliced
- ✓ 2½ cups tomatoes, finely chopped
- ✓ 1 teaspoon dried rosemary, crushed

Directions:
- ❖ In a large skillet, melt the coconut oil over medium heat and sauté the onion, celery and garlic for about 5 minutes.
- ❖ Add the rest of all ingredients and stir to combine.
- ❖ Increase heat to high and bring to a boil.
- ❖ Cook for about 10 minutes.

Ingredients:
- ✓ 1 teaspoon dried sage, crushed
- ✓ 1 teaspoon dried oregano, crushed
- ✓ Sea salt and freshly ground black pepper, to taste
- ✓ 2 cups of homemade vegetable broth
- ✓ 3-4 cups of alkaline water
- ✓ ¼ cup fresh parsley, chopped

- ❖ Reduce heat to medium and cook, covered for about 15 minutes.
- ❖ Uncover the pan and cook for about 15 minutes, stirring occasionally.
- ❖ Now, reduce the heat to low and simmer, covered for about 1 1/2 hours.
- ❖ Serve warm with a garnish of parsley.

Nutrition: Calories

43)   Tofu and bell pepper stew

Preparation time: 15 minutes   **Cooking time**: 15 minutes   **Servings**: 6

Ingredients:
- ✓ 2 tablespoons of garlic
- ✓ 1 jalapeño bell pepper, seeded and chopped
- ✓ 1 (16-ounce) can of roasted, rinsed, drained and chopped red peppers
- ✓ 2 cups of homemade vegetable broth
- ✓ 2 cups of alkaline water

Directions:
- ❖ In a food processor, add the garlic, jalapeño bell pepper and roasted red peppers and pulse until smooth.
- ❖ In a large skillet, add the pepper puree, broth and water over medium-high heat and bring to a boil.
- ❖ Add the peppers and tofu and stir to combine.

Ingredients:
- ✓ 1 medium green bell pepper, seeded and thinly sliced
- ✓ 1 medium red bell pepper, seeded and thinly sliced
- ✓ 1 (16-ounce) package of extra-firm tofu, drained and diced
- ✓ 10 ounces of frozen sprouts, thawed
- ✓ Sea salt and freshly ground black pepper, to taste

- ❖ Reduce the heat to medium and cook for about 5 minutes.
- ❖ Stir in the cabbage and cook for about 5 minutes.
- ❖ Add the salt and black pepper and remove from heat.
- ❖ Serve hot.

Nutrition: Calories

44)   Roasted Pumpkin Curry

Preparation time: 15 minutes   **Cooking time**: 35 minutes   **Servings**: 4

Ingredients:
- For the roasted squash:
- ✓ 1 medium-sized sugar pumpkin, peeled and cut into cubes
- ✓ Sea salt, to taste
- ✓ 1 teaspoon of olive oil
- For Curry:
- ✓ 1 teaspoon of olive oil
- ✓ 1 onion, chopped
- ✓ 1 tablespoon fresh ginger root, peeled and chopped

Directions:
- ❖ Preheat oven to 400 degrees F. Line a large baking sheet with baking paper.
- ❖ In a large bowl, add all the ingredients for the roasted squash and stir to coat well.
- ❖ Arrange the pumpkins on the prepared baking sheet in a single layer.
- ❖ Roast for about 20-25 minutes, turning once halfway through.

Nutrition: Calories

Ingredients:
- ✓ 1 tablespoon chopped garlic
- ✓ 1 cup unsweetened coconut milk
- ✓ 2 cups of vegetable broth
- ✓ 1 teaspoon of ground cumin
- ✓ ½ teaspoon ground turmeric
- ✓ Sea salt and freshly ground black pepper, to taste
- ✓ 1 tablespoon fresh lime juice
- ✓ 2 tablespoons fresh parsley, chopped
- ❖ Meanwhile, for the curry: in a large skillet, heat the oil over medium-high heat and sauté the onion for about 4-5 minutes.
- ❖ Add the ginger and garlic and sauté for about 1 minute.
- ❖ Add the coconut milk, broth, spices, salt and black pepper and bring to a boil.
- ❖ Reduce the heat to low and simmer for about 10 minutes.
- ❖ Add the roasted squash and simmer for another 10 minutes.
- ❖ Serve warm with a garnish of parsley.

45)   Lentils, vegetables and apple curry

Preparation time: 20 minutes   **Cooking time**: 1 hour and a half   **Servings**: 6

Ingredients:
- ✓ 8 cups of alkaline water
- ✓ ½ teaspoon ground turmeric
- ✓ 1 cup brown lentils
- ✓ 1 cup of red lentils
- ✓ 1 tablespoon of olive oil
- ✓ 1 large white onion, chopped
- ✓ 3 garlic cloves, minced
- ✓ 2 tomatoes, seeded and chopped

Directions:
- ❖ In a large skillet, add the water, turmeric and lentils over high heat and bring to a boil.
- ❖ Reduce heat to medium-low and simmer, covered for about 30 minutes.
- ❖ Drain the lentils, reserving 2½ cups of the cooking liquid.
- ❖ Meanwhile, in another large skillet, heat the oil over medium heat and sauté the onion for about 2-3 minutes.
- ❖ Add the garlic and sauté for about 1 minute.
- ❖ Add the tomatoes and cook for about 5 minutes.

Nutrition: Calories

Ingredients:
- ✓ ¼ teaspoon ground cloves
- ✓ 2 teaspoons of ground cumin
- ✓ 2 carrots, peeled and cut into pieces
- ✓ 2 potatoes, peeled and cut into pieces
- ✓ 2 cups pumpkin, peeled, seeded and cut into 1-inch cubes
- ✓ 1 granny smith apple, cored and chopped
- ✓ 2 cups fresh cabbage, hard ribs removed and chopped
- ✓ Sea salt and freshly ground black pepper, to taste
- ❖ Stir in the spices and cook for about 1 minute.
- ❖ Add the carrots, potatoes, squash, cooked lentils and reserved cooking liquid and bring to a gentle boil.
- ❖ Reduce heat to medium-low and simmer, covered for about 40-45 minutes or until desired doneness of vegetables.
- ❖ Add the apple and cabbage and simmer for about 15 minutes.
- ❖ Add the salt and black pepper and remove from heat.
- ❖ Serve hot.

46)   Curried red beans

Preparation time: 15 minutes   **Cooking time**: 25 minutes   **Servings**: 6

Ingredients:
- ✓ 4 tablespoons of olive oil
- ✓ 1 medium onion, finely chopped
- ✓ 2 garlic cloves, minced
- ✓ 2 tablespoons of fresh ginger root, peeled and chopped
- ✓ 1 teaspoon of ground coriander
- ✓ 1 teaspoon of ground cumin
- ✓ ½ teaspoon ground turmeric

Directions:
- ❖ In a large skillet, heat the oil over medium heat and sauté the onion, garlic and ginger for about 6-8 minutes.
- ❖ Stir in the spices and cook for about 1-2 minutes.

Nutrition: Calories

Ingredients:
- ✓ ¼ teaspoon cayenne pepper
- ✓ Sea salt and freshly ground black pepper, to taste
- ✓ 2 large plum tomatoes, finely chopped
- ✓ 3 cups of cooked red beans
- ✓ 2 cups of alkaline water
- ✓ ¼ cup fresh parsley, chopped

- ❖ Add the tomatoes, beans and water and bring to a boil over high heat.
- ❖ Reduce heat to medium and simmer for 10-15 minutes or until desired thickness.
- ❖ Serve warm with a garnish of parsley.

47) Lentil and Carrot Chili

Preparation time: 15 minutes   **Cooking time:** 2 hours and 40 minutes   **Servings: 8**

Ingredients:
- ✓ 2 teaspoons of olive oil
- ✓ 1 large onion, chopped
- ✓ 3 medium carrots, peeled and chopped
- ✓ 4 celery stalks, chopped
- ✓ 2 garlic cloves, minced
- ✓ • 1 jalapeño bell pepper, seeded and chopped
- ✓ ½ tablespoon dried thyme, crushed
- ✓ 1 tablespoon of chipotle chili powder

Ingredients:
- ✓ ½ tablespoon of cayenne pepper
- ✓ 1½ tablespoons ground coriander
- ✓ 1½ tablespoons of ground cumin
- ✓ 1 teaspoon ground turmeric
- ✓ Sea salt and freshly ground black pepper, to taste
- ✓ 1 pound red lentils, rinsed
- ✓ 8 cups of homemade vegetable broth
- ✓ ½ cup shallots, chopped

Directions:
- ❖ In a large skillet, heat the oil over medium heat and sauté the onion, carrot and celery for about 5 minutes.
- ❖ Add the garlic, jalapeño pepper, thyme and spices and sauté for about 1 minute.

- ❖ Add the lentils and broth and bring to a boil.
- ❖ Reduce heat to low and simmer, covered for about 2-2½ hours.
- ❖ Remove from heat and serve hot with a scallion garnish.

Nutrition: Calories

48) Black beans with chilli

Preparation time: 15 minutes   **Cooking time:** 2 hours and 5 minutes   **Servings: 5**

Ingredients:
- ✓ 2 tablespoons of olive oil
- ✓ 1 onion, chopped
- ✓ 1 large green bell pepper, seeded and sliced
- ✓ 4 garlic cloves, minced
- ✓ 2 jalapeño peppers, sliced
- ✓ 1 teaspoon of ground cumin
- ✓ 1 teaspoon of cayenne pepper

Ingredients:
- ✓ 1 tablespoon of red chili powder
- ✓ 1 teaspoon of paprika
- ✓ 2 cups of tomatoes, finely chopped
- ✓ 4 cups of cooked black beans
- ✓ 2 cups of homemade vegetable broth
- ✓ Sea salt and freshly ground black pepper, to taste
- ✓ ¼ cup fresh parsley, chopped

Directions:
- ❖ In a large skillet, heat the oil over medium-high heat and sauté the onion and peppers for 3-4 minutes.
- ❖ Add the garlic, jalapeño peppers and spices and sauté for about 1 minute.
- ❖ Add the remaining ingredients and bring to a boil.

- ❖ Reduce heat to medium-low and simmer, covered for about 1½-2 hours.
- ❖ Season with the salt and black pepper and remove from heat.
- ❖ Serve warm with a garnish of parsley.

Nutrition: Calories

49) Cook mixed vegetables

Preparation time: 15 minutes   **Cooking time:** 20 minutes   **Servings: 4**

Ingredients:
- ✓ 1 small zucchini, chopped
- ✓ 1 small summer squash, chopped
- ✓ 1 diced eggplant
- ✓ 1 red bell pepper, seeded and diced
- ✓ 1 green bell pepper, seeded and diced

Ingredients:
- ✓ 1 onion, thinly sliced
- ✓ 1 tablespoon of pure maple syrup
- ✓ 2 tablespoons of olive oil
- ✓ Sea salt and freshly ground black pepper, to taste

Directions:
- ❖ Preheat oven to 375 degrees F. Lightly grease a large baking dish.
- ❖ In a large bowl, add all ingredients and mix well.

- ❖ Transfer the vegetable mixture to the prepared baking dish.
- ❖ Bake for about 15-20 minutes.
- ❖ Remove from oven and serve immediately.

Nutrition: Calories

50) Vegetarian Ratatouille

Preparation time: 20 minutes   **Cooking time:** 45 minutes   **Servings: 4**

Ingredients:
- ✓ 6 ounces of homemade tomato paste
- ✓ 3 tablespoons of olive oil, divided by
- ✓ ½ onion, chopped
- ✓ 3 tablespoons minced garlic
- ✓ Sea salt and freshly ground black pepper, to taste

Ingredients:
- ✓ 1 yellow pumpkin, cut in thin circles
- ✓ 1 eggplant, cut into thin circles
- ✓ 1 red bell pepper, with seeds and cut into thin rounds
- ✓ 1 yellow bell pepper, with seeds and cut into thin rounds
- ✓ 1 tablespoon fresh thyme leaves, chopped

✓ 1 zucchini, cut into thin circles   ✓ 1 tablespoon fresh lemon juice

Directions:
❖ Preheat the oven to 375 degrees F.
❖ In a bowl, add tomato paste, 1 tablespoon oil, onion, garlic, salt and black pepper and mix well.
❖ In the bottom of a 10x10-inch baking dish, spread tomato paste mixture evenly.
❖ Arrange the vegetable slices alternately, starting at the outer edge of the pan and working concentrically toward the center.

Nutrition: Calories

❖ Drizzle the vegetables with the remaining oil and sprinkle with salt and black pepper, followed by the thyme.
❖ Arrange a piece of parchment paper over the vegetables.
❖ Bake for about 45 minutes.
❖ Remove from oven and serve hot.

51) Quinoa with vegetables

Preparation time: 15 minutes   **Cooking time:** 26 minutes   **Servings: 4**

Ingredients:
   For roasted mushrooms:
✓ 2 cups of small fresh Baby Bella mushrooms
✓ 1 tablespoon of olive oil
✓ Sea salt, to taste
   For the quinoa:
✓ 2 cups of alkaline water
✓ 1 cup red quinoa, rinsed
✓ 2 tablespoons fresh parsley, chopped

Directions:
❖ Preheat oven to 425 degrees F. Line a large rimmed baking sheet with parchment paper.
❖ In a bowl, add the mushrooms, oil and salt and stir to coat well.
❖ Arrange the mushrooms on the prepared baking sheet in a single layer.
❖ Roast for about 15-18 minutes, tossing once halfway through cooking.
❖ Meanwhile, for the quinoa: in a skillet, add the water and quinoa over medium-high heat and bring to a boil.
❖ Reduce the heat to low and simmer, covered for about 15-20 minutes or until all the liquid is absorbed.
❖ Remove from heat and set pan aside, covered for about 5 minutes.
❖ Uncover the pan and with a fork, stir in the quinoa.

Nutrition: Calories

Ingredients:
✓ 1 garlic clove chopped
✓ 1 tablespoon of olive oil
✓ 2 teaspoons of fresh lemon juice
✓ Sea salt and freshly ground black pepper, to taste
   For the broccoli:
✓ 1 cup of broccoli florets
✓ 2 tablespoons of olive oil

❖ Stir in the parsley, garlic, oil, lemon juice, salt and black pepper and set aside to cool completely.
❖ Meanwhile, for the broccoli: in a pot of water, arrange a steamer basket and bring to a boil.
❖ Place the broccoli florets in the basket of the steamer and steam, covered for about 5-6 minutes.
❖ Drain broccoli florets well.
❖ Transfer the broccoli florets to the bowl with the quinoa and mushrooms and stir to combine.
❖ Drizzle with the oil and serve immediately.

52) Lentils with cabbage

Preparation time: 15 minutes   **Cooking time:** 20 minutes   **Servings: 6**

Ingredients:
✓ 1½ cups of red lentils
✓ 1½ cups homemade vegetable broth
✓ 1½ tablespoons of olive oil
✓ ½ cup onion, chopped
✓ 1 teaspoon fresh ginger, chopped

Directions:
❖ In a skillet, add the broth and lentils over medium-high heat and bring to a boil.
❖ Reduce heat and simmer, covered for about 20 minutes or until almost all liquid is absorbed.
❖ Remove from heat and set aside covered.

Nutrition: Calories

Ingredients:
✓ 2 garlic cloves, minced
✓ 1½ cups tomato, chopped
✓ 6 cups fresh cabbage, hard ribs removed and chopped
✓ Sea salt and ground black pepper, to taste

❖ Meanwhile, in a large skillet, heat the oil over medium heat and sauté the onion for about 5-6 minutes.
❖ Add the ginger and garlic and sauté for about 1 minute.
❖ Add the tomatoes and cabbage and cook for about 4-5 minutes.
❖ Add the lentils, salt and black pepper and remove from heat.
❖ Remove from heat and serve hot.

53)   Lentils with tomatoes

Preparation time: 15 minutes   **Cooking time:** 55 minutes   **Servings: 4**

Ingredients:
- ✓ For the tomato puree:
- ✓ 1 cup tomatoes, chopped
- ✓ 1 garlic clove, minced
- ✓ 1 green chilli chopped
- ✓ ¼ cup alkaline water
-    For the lentils:
- ✓ 1 cup of red lentils
- ✓ 3 cups of alkaline water

Directions:
- ❖ To tomato paste in a blender, add all ingredients and pulse until it forms a smooth puree. Set aside.
- ❖ In a large skillet, add 3 cups of water and the lentils over high heat and bring to a boil.
- ❖ Reduce heat to medium-low and simmer, covered for about 15-20 minutes or until quite tender.
- ❖ Drain lentils well.

Nutrition: Calories

Ingredients:
- ✓ 1 tablespoon of olive oil
- ✓ ½ medium white onion, chopped
- ✓ ½ teaspoon of ground cumin
- ✓ ½ teaspoon of cayenne pepper
- ✓ ¼ teaspoon ground turmeric
- ✓ ¼ cup tomato, chopped
- ✓ ¼ cup fresh parsley leaves, chopped

- ❖ In a large skillet, heat the oil over medium heat and sauté the onion for about 6-7 minutes.
- ❖ Add the spices and sauté for about 1 minute.
- ❖ Add the tomato puree and cook, stirring for about 5-7 minutes.
- ❖ Stir in lentils and cook for about 4-5 minutes or until desired degree of doneness.
- ❖ Stir in chopped tomato and immediately remove from heat.
- ❖   Serve warm with a garnish of parsley.

54)   Spicy baked beans

Preparation time: 15 minutes   **Cooking time:** 2 hours and 5 minutes   **Servings: 4**

Ingredients:
- ✓ ½ pound of dried red beans, soaked overnight and drained
- ✓ 1¼ tablespoons of olive oil
- ✓ 1 small yellow onion, chopped
- ✓ 4 garlic cloves, minced
- ✓ 1 teaspoon dried thyme, crushed
- ✓ ½ teaspoon of ground cumin
- ✓ ½ teaspoon of red pepper flakes, crushed

Directions:
- ❖ In a large pot of boiling water, add the beans and bring to a boil.
- ❖ Reduce heat to low and cook, covered for about 1 hour.
- ❖ Remove from heat and drain beans well.
- ❖ Preheat the oven to 325 degrees F.
- ❖ In a large ovenproof skillet, heat the oil over medium heat and sauté the onion for about 4 minutes.

Nutrition: Calories

Ingredients:
- ✓ ¼ teaspoon of smoked paprika
- ✓ 1 tablespoon fresh lemon juice
- ✓ 1 cup of homemade tomato sauce
- ✓ 1 cup of homemade vegetable broth
- ✓ Sea salt and freshly ground black pepper, to taste

- ❖ Add the garlic, thyme and spices and sauté for about 1 minute.
- ❖ Add the cooked beans and other ingredients and immediately remove from heat.
- ❖ Cover the pan and bake for about 1 hour.
- ❖ Remove from oven and serve hot.

55)   Chickpeas with pumpkin

Preparation time: 20 minutes   **Cooking time:** 35 minutes   **Servings: 4**

Ingredients:
- ✓ 1 tablespoon of olive oil
- ✓ 1 onion, chopped
- ✓ 2 garlic cloves, minced
- ✓ 1 green chili pepper, seedless and finely chopped
- ✓ 1 teaspoon of ground cumin
- ✓ ½ teaspoon of ground coriander
- ✓ 1 teaspoon of red chili powder

Directions:
- ❖ In a large skillet, heat the oil over medium-high heat and sauté the onion for about 5-7 minutes.
- ❖ Add the garlic, green chiles and spices and sauté for about 1 minute.
- ❖ Add tomatoes and cook for 2-3 minutes, mashing with the back of a spoon.

Nutrition: Calories

Ingredients:
- ✓ 2 cups fresh tomatoes, finely chopped
- ✓ 2 pounds of pumpkin, peeled and diced
- ✓ 2 cups of homemade vegetable broth
- ✓ 2 cups of cooked chickpeas
- ✓ 2 tablespoons fresh lemon juice
- ✓ Sea salt and freshly ground black pepper, to taste
- ✓ 2 tablespoons fresh parsley leaves, chopped
- ❖ Add the squash and cook for about 3-4 minutes, stirring occasionally.
- ❖ Add the broth and bring to a boil.
- ❖ Reduce the heat to low and simmer for about 10 minutes.
- ❖ Stir in the chickpeas and simmer for about 10 minutes.
- ❖ Add the lemon juice, salt and black pepper and remove from heat.
- ❖ Serve warm with a garnish of parsley.

56) Chickpeas with cabbage

Preparation time: 15 minutes   **Cooking time**: 18 minutes   **Servings**: 6

Ingredients:
- ✓ 2 tablespoons of olive oil
- ✓ 1 medium onion, chopped
- ✓ 4 garlic cloves, minced
- ✓ 1 teaspoon dried thyme, crushed
- ✓ 1 teaspoon dried oregano, crushed
- ✓ ½ teaspoon of paprika
- ✓ 1 cup of tomato, finely chopped

Ingredients:
- ✓ 2 ½ cups cooked chickpeas
- ✓ 4 cups fresh cabbage, hard ribs removed and chopped
- ✓ 2 tablespoons of alkaline water
- ✓ 2 tablespoons fresh lemon juice
- ✓ Sea salt and freshly ground black pepper, to taste
- ✓ 3 tablespoons fresh basil, chopped

Directions:
- ❖ In a large skillet, heat the oil over medium heat and sauté the onion for about 8-9 minutes.
- ❖ Add the garlic, herbs and paprika and sauté for about 1 minute.
- ❖ Add the cabbage and water and cook for about 2-3 minutes.

- ❖ Add the tomatoes and chickpeas and cook for about 3-5 minutes.
- ❖ Add the lemon juice, salt and black pepper and remove from heat.
- ❖ Serve warm with the basil garnish.

Nutrition: Calories

57) Stuffed cabbage rolls

Preparation time: 15 minutes   **Cooking time**: 15 minutes   **Servings**: 4

Ingredients:
  For filling:
- ✓ 1½ cups fresh button mushrooms, chopped
- ✓ 3¼ cups zucchini, chopped
- ✓ 1 cup red bell bell pepper, seeded and chopped
- ✓ 1 cup green bell pepper, seeded and chopped
- ✓ ½ teaspoon dried thyme, crushed
- ✓ ½ teaspoon dried marjoram, crushed
- ✓ ½ teaspoon dried basil, crushed

Ingredients:
- ✓ Sea salt and freshly ground black pepper, to taste
- ✓ ½ cup homemade vegetable broth
- ✓ 2 teaspoons of fresh lemon juice
  For rolls:
- ✓ 8 large cabbage leaves, rinsed
- ✓ 8 ounces of homemade tomato sauce
- ✓ 3 tablespoons fresh parsley, chopped

Directions:
- ❖ Preheat oven to 400 degrees F. Lightly grease a 13x9-inch casserole dish.
- ❖ For the filling: in a large skillet, add all ingredients except lemon juice over medium heat and bring to a boil.
- ❖ Reduce heat to low and simmer, covered for about 5 minutes.
- ❖ Remove from heat and set aside for about 5 minutes.
- ❖ Add the lemon juice and stir to combine.
- ❖ Meanwhile, for the rolls: in a large pot of boiling water, add the cabbage leaves and boil for about 2-4 minutes.
- ❖ Drain the cabbage leaves well.
- ❖ Thoroughly dry each cabbage leaf with paper towels.
- ❖ Arrange the cabbage leaves on a smooth surface.
- ❖ Using a knife, make a V-shaped cut in each leaf by cutting through the thick vein.

- ❖ Carefully overlap the cut ends of each leaf.
- ❖ Place the filling mixture evenly on each leaf and fold in the sides.
- ❖ Then, roll up each leaf to seal in the filling and then, secure each leaf with toothpicks.
- ❖ In the bottom of the prepared casserole dish, place 1/3 cup of the tomato sauce evenly.
- ❖ Arrange cabbage rolls on top of sauce in a single layer and top with remaining sauce evenly.
- ❖ Cover the casserole dish and cook for about 15 minutes.
- ❖ Remove from oven and set aside, uncovered for about 5 minutes.
- ❖ Serve warm with a garnish of parsley.

Nutrition: Calories

58) Green beans and mushrooms in casserole

Preparation time: 20 minutes   **Cooking time**: 20 minutes   **Servings**: 6

Ingredients:
For the onion slices:
- ✓ ½ cup yellow onion, very thinly sliced
- ✓ ¼ cup almond flour
- ✓ 1/8 teaspoon of garlic powder
- ✓ Sea salt and freshly ground black pepper, to taste
For the casserole:
- ✓ 1 pound fresh green beans, chopped
- ✓ 1 tablespoon of olive oil

Directions:
- ❖ Preheat the oven to 350 degrees F.
- ❖ For the onion slices: in a bowl, place all ingredients and mix to coat well.
- ❖ Arrange the onion slices on a large baking sheet in a single layer and set aside.
- ❖ For the casserole: in a pot of boiling salted water, add the green beans and cook for about 5 minutes.
- ❖ Drain green beans and transfer to a bowl of ice water.
- ❖ Again, drain well and transfer to a large bowl. Set aside.
- ❖ In a large skillet, heat the oil over medium-high heat and sauté the mushrooms, onion, garlic powder, salt and black pepper for about 2-3 minutes.

Nutrition: Calories

Ingredients:
- ✓ 8 ounces fresh cremini mushrooms, sliced
- ✓ ½ cup yellow onion, thinly sliced
- ✓ 1/8 teaspoon of garlic powder
- ✓ Sea salt and freshly ground black pepper, to taste
- ✓ 1 teaspoon fresh thyme, chopped
- ✓ ½ cup homemade vegetable broth
- ✓ ½ cup of coconut cream

- ❖ Stir in the thyme and broth and cook for about 3-5 minutes or until all the liquid is absorbed.
- ❖ Remove from heat and transfer the mushroom mixture to the bowl with the green beans.
- ❖ Add the coconut cream and stir to combine well.
- ❖ Transfer the mixture to a 10-inch casserole dish.
- ❖ Place the casserole dish and onion slice pan in the oven.
- ❖ Bake for about 15-17 minutes.
- ❖ Remove the pan and sheet from the oven and let cool for about 5 minutes before serving.
- ❖ Top the casserole with the crispy onion slices evenly.
- ❖ Cut into 6 equal-sized portions and serve.

59) Meatloaf of wild rice and lentils

Preparation time: 20 minutes   **Cooking time**: 1 hour and 50 minutes   **Servings**: 8

Ingredients:
- ✓ 1¾ cups plus 2 tablespoons of alkaline water, divided
- ✓ ½ cup wild rice
- ✓ ½ cup of brown lentils
- ✓ Pinch of sea salt
- ✓ ½ teaspoon of sodium-free Italian seasoning
- ✓ 1 medium yellow onion, chopped
- ✓ 1 celery stalk, chopped
- ✓ 6 cremini mushrooms, chopped

Directions:
- ❖ In a saucepan, add 1¾ cups water, the rice, lentils, salt and Italian seasoning and bring to a boil over medium-high heat.
- ❖ Reduce the heat to low and simmer covered for about 45 minutes.
- ❖ Remove from heat and set aside, covered for at least 10 minutes.
- ❖ Preheat oven to 350 degrees F. Line a 9x5-inch baking dish with baking paper.
- ❖ In a skillet, heat the remaining water over medium heat and sauté the onion, celery, mushrooms and garlic for about 4-5 minutes.
- ❖ Remove from heat and allow to cool slightly.
- ❖ In a large bowl, add the oats, pecans, tomato sauce and fresh herbs and stir until well combined.

Nutrition: Calories

Ingredients:
- ✓ 4 garlic cloves, minced
- ✓ ¾ cup rolled oats
- ✓ ½ cup pecans, finely chopped
- ✓ ¾ cup of homemade tomato sauce
- ✓ ½ teaspoon of red pepper flakes, crushed
- ✓ 1 teaspoon fresh rosemary, chopped
- ✓ 2 teaspoons fresh thyme, chopped

- ❖ Combine the rice mixture and vegetable mixture with the oat mixture and mix well.
- ❖ In a blender, add the mixture and pulse until it forms a chunky mixture.
- ❖ Transfer the mixture to the prepared baking dish evenly.
- ❖ With a piece of foil, cover the pan and bake for about 40 minutes.
- ❖ Uncover and bake for about 15-20 minutes more or until the top turns golden brown.
- ❖ Remove from oven and set aside for about 5-10 minutes before slicing.
- ❖ Cut into slices of desired size and serve

60) Vegetable soup and spelt noodles

Preparation time: 5 minutes   **Cooking time:** 12 minutes   **Servings: 2**

Ingredients:
- ✓ ½ onion, peeled, cut into cubes
- ✓ ½ green bell pepper, chopped
- ✓ ½ zucchini, grated
- ✓ 4 ounces (113 g) sliced mushrooms, chopped
- ✓ ½ cup of cherry tomatoes
- ✓ ¼ cup of basil leaves

Directions:
- ❖ Take a medium saucepan, put it over medium heat, add the oil and when hot, add the onion and then cook for 3 minutes or more until tender.
- ❖ Add the cherry tomatoes, bell bell pepper and mushrooms, stir until combined and continue cooking for 3 minutes until soft.
- ❖ Add the grated zucchini, season with salt, cayenne pepper, pour in the water and bring the mixture to a boil.

Nutrition: Calories

Ingredients:
- ✓ 1 package of spelt tagliatelle, cooked
- ✓ ¼ teaspoon salt
- ✓ ⅛ teaspoon of cayenne pepper
- ✓ ½ key lime, squeezed
- ✓ 1 tablespoon of grape oil
- ✓ 2 cups of spring water
- ❖ Then, turn the heat down to low, add the cooked noodles and simmer the soup for 5 minutes.
- ❖ When finished, pour soup into two bowls, top with basil leaves, drizzle with lime juice and serve.

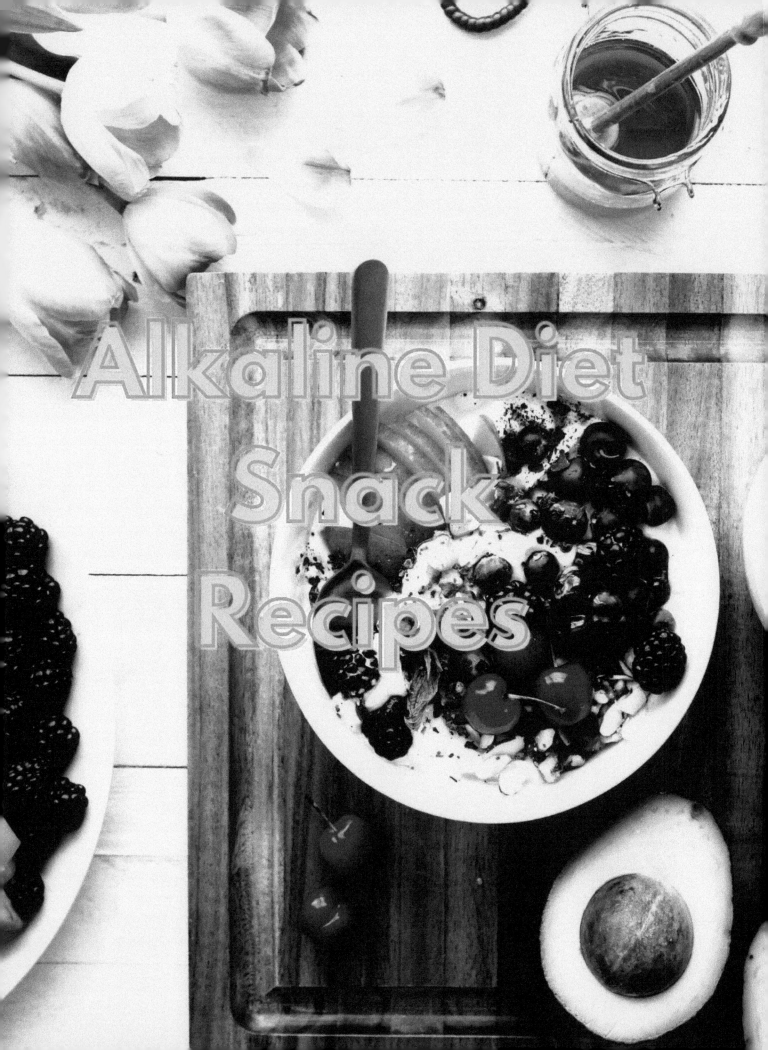

61)   Quinoa Salad

Preparation time: **Cooking time**:   **Servings: 2**

Ingredients:
- ✓ 1 cup quinoa, cooked
- ✓ 1 garlic clove, minced
- ✓ 1 cucumber, chopped
- ✓ 1 cup of fresh arugula leaves
- ✓ 1 red bell pepper, chopped
- ✓ 1 large avocado, peeled, pitted and diced

Directions:
- ❖ Just combine all the ingredients in a large salad bowl.

Nutrition: Calories

Ingredients:
- ✓ 2 tablespoons of chia seeds (optional)
- ✓ 2 tablespoons of olive oil
- ✓ 2 tablespoons of coconut milk (I think)
- ✓ Himalayan salt and black pepper to taste
- ✓ Juice of 1 lime or lemon

- ❖ Mix well and drizzle with olive oil, coconut milk and lemon juice.
- ❖ Enjoy!

62)   Almonds with sautéed vegetables

Preparation time: **Cooking time**:   **Servings: 4**

Ingredients:
- ✓ Young beans, 150g
- ✓ Broccoli flower, 4
- ✓ Oregano and cumin, ½ teaspoon
- ✓ Lemon juice (fresh), 3 tablespoons
- ✓ Garlic clove (finely chopped), 1

Directions:
- ❖ Add broccoli, beans and other vegetables to a large skillet and fry until beans and broccoli turn dark green.
- ❖ Make sure the vegetables are crispy as well.
- ❖ Now add the chopped garlic and onion, sauté and stir for a few minutes.

Nutrition: Calories

Ingredients:
- ✓ Cauliflower, 1 cup
- ✓ Olive oil (cold pressed), 4 tablespoons
- ✓ Pepper and salt to taste
- ✓ Some soaked almonds (sliced), for garnish
- ✓ Yellow onion, 1
- ❖ Then, put the dressing together.
- ❖ Take a small bowl, add the lemon juice, oregano, cumin and oil and mix well.
- ❖ Add some vegetables, stir slowly and taste for pepper and salt.
- ❖ Finally, use the sliced almonds for garnish.
- ❖ Serve.

63)   Alkaline Sweet Potato Mash

Preparation time: **Cooking time**:   **Servings: 3-4**

Ingredients:
- ✓ Sea salt, 1 tablespoon
- ✓ Curry powder, ½ tablespoon
- ✓ Sweet potatoes (large), 6

Directions:
- ❖ First, get a large mixing bowl.
- ❖ Wash and cut the sweet potatoes and add them to the cooking pot and cook for about twenty minutes.

Nutrition: Calories

Ingredients:
- ✓ Coconut milk (fresh), 1 ½ - 2 cups
- ✓ Extra virgin olive oil (cold pressed), 1 tablespoon
- ✓ Pepper, 1 pinch

- ❖ Then, remove the sweet potatoes and mash them to your desired consistency.
- ❖ Finally, all you have to do is add the remaining ingredients and serve.

64)   Mediterranean peppers

Preparation time: **Cooking time**:   **Servings: 2**

Ingredients:
- ✓ Oregano, 1 teaspoon
- ✓ Garlic cloves (crushed), 2
- ✓ Fresh parsley (chopped), 2 tablespoons
- ✓ Vegetable broth (no yeast), 1 cup
- ✓ Provincial herbs, 1 teaspoon

Directions:
- ❖ Heat the olive oil in a skillet over medium heat, add the bell bell pepper and onions and stir.
- ❖ Add the garlic and stir.

Ingredients:
- ✓ Red bell pepper (sliced) 2 + Yellow bell pepper (sliced) 2
- ✓ Red onions (thinly sliced), 2 medium-sized
- ✓ Extra virgin olive oil (cold pressed), 2 tablespoons
- ✓ Salt and pepper to taste

- ❖ Then, add the vegetable stock and season with parsley and herbs, as well as pepper and salt to taste.
- ❖ Cover the pan and let it cook for fourteen to fifteen minutes.
- ❖ Serve.

65)   Tomato and avocado sauce with potatoes

Preparation time: **Cooking time:**   **Servings: 3**

Ingredients:
- ✓ Red onion 1
- ✓ 2 Tomatoes
- ✓ ½ - 1 lemon (squeezed)
- ✓ Chives (fresh and chopped), 1 teaspoon
- ✓ Parsley (fresh and chopped), 1 teaspoon

Directions:
- ❖ Take a pan and cook the potatoes in salted water, (cook the potatoes with the skin intact).
- ❖ Next, peel the avocado, toss it in a bowl and mash it with a fork.

Nutrition: Calories

Ingredients:
- ✓ Cayenne pepper, ½ teaspoon
- ✓ Avocado (ripe), 2
- ✓ Waxy potatoes (medium size), 6
- ✓ Saltwater
- ✓ Pepper and salt
- ❖ Now, dice the onion and tomatoes, add them to the bowl along with the parsley, chives and cayenne.
- ❖ Mix well and season with pepper, lemon juice and salt.
- ❖ Serve along with the potatoes.

66)   Alkaline beans and coconut

Preparation time: **Cooking time:**   **Servings: 4**

Ingredients:
- ✓ Ground cumin, ½ teaspoon
- ✓ Red chili pepper (chopped), 1-2
- ✓ Coconut milk (fresh), 3 tablespoons
- ✓ Dry flaked coconut, 1 tablespoon
- ✓ Garlic (chopped), 2 cloves
- ✓ Cayenne pepper, 1 pinch

Directions:
- ❖ Heat the oil in a skillet and add the beans, cumin, garlic, ginger and glaze and sauté for about six minutes.

Nutrition: Calories

Ingredients:
- ✓ Sea salt, 1 pinch
- ✓ Extra virgin olive oil (cold pressed), 3 tablespoons
- ✓ Fresh herbs of your choice, 1 teaspoon
- ✓ One (1) pound of green beans, cut into 1-inch pieces
- ✓ Fresh ginger (chopped), ½ teaspoon

- ❖ Add the coconut flakes and oil and sauté until the milk is fully cooked (this may take three or four minutes).
- ❖ Season with pepper, salt and herbs to taste. Serve.

67)   Alkalized vegetable lasagna

Preparation time: **Cooking time:**   **Servings: 1**

Ingredients:
- ✓ Parsley root, 1
- ✓ Leek (small), 1
- ✓ Radish (small), 1
- ✓ Corn salad, 1
- ✓ Tomatoes (large), 3
- ✓ Garlic, 1 clove

Directions:
- ❖ Take a blender and add the lemon juice, garlic clove and avocado.
- ❖ Cut the bell bell pepper into thin strips, cut the leek into thin rings and finely grate the parsley root and radish. When you are done, mix everything with the avocado cream.

Nutrition: Calories

Ingredients:
- ✓ Avocado (soft), 2
- ✓ Lemon (squeezed), 1-2
- ✓ Arugula, 1
- ✓ Parsley (few)
- ✓ Red bell pepper, 1

- ❖ Let's start with the first layer of the lasagna.
- ❖ Deposit corn salad in a casserole dish, add avocado spread well.
- ❖ For the second layer, add the sliced tomatoes.
- ❖ Finally, add the arugula and parsley for the final layer.
- ❖ Serve.

68)   Aloo Gobi

Preparation time: **Cooking time**:   **Servings: 1 bowl**

Ingredients:
- ✓ Cauliflower, 750g
- ✓ Fresh ginger, 20g
- ✓ Large onions, 2
- ✓ Mint, 1/3 cup
- ✓ Turmeric, 2 teaspoons
- ✓ Diced tomatoes, 400g
- ✓ Fresh garlic, 2 cloves
- ✓ Cayenne pepper, 2 teaspoons

Directions:
- ❖ Blend the chili, garlic and ginger.
- ❖ Fry oil in a wok for three minutes and add onion until golden brown.
- ❖ Add ground pasta and sauté for a few seconds, then add; garam masala, chili, turmeric, tomatoes and salt.

Nutrition: Calories

Ingredients:
- ✓ Cilantro/coriander leaves, 1/3 cup
- ✓ Large potatoes, 4
- ✓ Garam masala, 2 teaspoons
- ✓ Green chilli, 4
- ✓ Water, 3 cups
- ✓ Extra virgin olive oil (cold pressed), 125 ml
- ✓ Salt to taste

- ❖ Cook for about five minutes and add all other ingredients.
- ❖ Stir for three minutes and add the water.
- ❖ Cook until sauce is thick.
- ❖ Serve with Basmati rice or as a side dish.

69)   Chocolate Crunch Bars

Preparation time: 3 hours   **Cooking time**: 5 minutes   **Servings: 4**

Ingredients:
- ✓ 1 1/2 cups sugar-free chocolate chips
- ✓ 1 cup of nut butter
- ✓ Stevia for taste

Directions:
- ❖ Prepare an 8-inch baking dish with baking paper.
- ❖ Mix chips chocolate with butter, coconut oil and sweetener in a bowl.
- ❖ Melt in the microwave for 2 to 3 minutes until melted.

Ingredients:
- ✓ 1/4 cup of coconut oil
- ✓ 3 cups pecans, chopped

- ❖ Add the nut and nuts. Stir gently.
- ❖ Put this wand in the oven and then it won't open anymore.
- ❖ Refrigerate for 2 to 3 hours.
- ❖ Slice and serve.

Nutrition: Calories 316 Fat: 30.9g. Carbs: 8.3g. Protein: 6.4g. Fiber: 3.8g.

70)   Nut Butter Bars

Preparation time: 40 minutes.   **Cooking time:** 10 minutes.   **Servings: 6**

Ingredients:
- ✓ 3/4 cup of walnut flour
- ✓ 2 ounces of nut butter
- ✓ 1/4 cup Swerve

Directions:
- ❖ Combine all the ingredients for best results.
- ❖ Transfer contents to a small 6-inch baking dish. Press down firmly.

Ingredients:
- ✓ 1/2 wooden walnut
- ✓ 1/2 teaspoon vanilla

- ❖ Refrigerate for 30 minutes.
- ❖ Cut into slices and serve.

Nutrition: Calories 214 Fat: 19g. Carbs: 6.5g. Protein: 6.5g. Fiber: 2.1g.

71)   Homemade Protein Bar

Preparation time: 5 mnutes   **Cooking time:** 10 minutes   **Servings: 4**

Ingredients:
- ✓ 1 knob of butter
- ✓ 4 tablespoons of coconut oil
- ✓ 2 scoops of vanilla protein

Directions:
- ❖ Mix coconut oil with butter, protein, stevia and salt in a dish.
- ❖ Mix cinnamon and chocolate chips.

Ingredients:
- ✓ To taste, ½ teaspoon of sea salt Optional Ingredients:
- ✓ 1 teaspoon cinnamon

- ❖ Presss the dough is firmly and freeze until firmed.
- ❖ Cut the crust into small bars.
- ❖ Serve and enjoy.

Nutrition: Calories 179 Fat: 15.7g. Carbohydrates: 4.8g. Protein: 5.6g. Fiber: 0.8g.

72)   Shortbread Coookies

Preparation time: 10 minutes   **Cooking time**: 1 hour and 10 minutes   **Servings: 6**

Ingredients:
- ✓ 2 1/2 cups coconut flour
- ✓ 6 tablespoons of nut butter

Directions:
- ❖ Preheat our oven to 350 degrees.
- ❖ Place on a cookie sheet with the parchment paper.
- ❖ Beat the butter with the erythritol until fluffy.
- ❖ Add the vanilla essence and coconut flour.

Ingredients:
- ✓ 1/2 cup erythritol
- ✓ 1 teaspoon of vanilla essence

- ❖ Mix everything together until crumbly.
- ❖ Spoon out a tablespoon of cookie dough onto the cookie sheet.
- ❖ Add more dough to make a stack.
- ❖ Bake for 15 minutes until golden brown.
- ❖ Serve.

Nutrition: Calories 288 Fat: 25.3g. Carbohydrates: 9.6g. Protein: 7.6g. Fiber: 3.8g.

73)   Coconut cookies Chip

Preparation time: 10 minutes   **Cooking time**: 15 minutes   **Servings: 4**

Ingredients:
- ✓ 1 cup of walnut flour
- ✓ ½ cup cacao nibs
- ✓ ½ cup coconut flakes, unsweetened
- ✓ 1/3 cup erythritol
- ✓ ½ cup nut butter

Directions:
- ❖ Prepare the oven for 350 degrees F.
- ❖ Layer a cookie sheet with parchment paper.
- ❖ Add and combine all ingredients dry in a glass bowl.
- ❖ Coconut milk, coconut milk, vanilla, stevia and peanut butter.
- ❖ Beating well compared to stir in the battery. Mix well.

Ingredients:
- ✓ ¼ cup peanut launcher, more than once
- ✓ ¼ cup of coconut milk
- ✓ Stevia, to taste
- ✓ ¼ teaspoon of sea salt

- ❖ Spoon out a tablespoon of cookie dough on the cooookie sheet.
- ❖ Add more dough to make 16 coookies.
- ❖ Fluctuate each cookie using your fingers.
- ❖ Water for 25 minutes until dawn.
- ❖ Let them rest for 15 minutes.
- ❖ Serve.

Nutrition: Calories 192 Fat: 17.44g. Carbohydrates: 2.2g. Protein: 4.7g. Fiber: 2.1g.

74)   Coconut Cookies

Preparation time: 10 mnutes   **Cooking time**: 20 minutes   **Servings: 6**

Ingredients:
- ✓ 6 tablespoons coconut flour
- ✓ ¾ teaspoons baking powder
- ✓ 1/8 teaspoon sea salt
- ✓ 3 tablespoons of nut butter

Directions:
- ❖ Preheat our oven to 375 degrees F. Layer a cookie sheet with parchment.
- ❖ Place all wet ingredients in a blender. Blend all the mixture in a blender.
- ❖ Add the wet mixture and mix well until used up.

Ingredients:
- ✓ 1/6 cup coconut oil
- ✓ 6 tablespoon data sugar
- ✓ 1/3 cup coco nut milk
- ✓ 1/2 teaspoon vanilla essence

- ❖ Place a spoonful of dough cookie on the cookie sheet.
- ❖ Add a little more butter to make many coookies. Bake until golden brown (about 10 minutes). We'll see.

Nutrition: Calories 151 Fat: 13.4g. Carbs: 6.4g. Protein: 4.2g. Fiber: 4.8g

75)   Berry Mousse

Preparation time: 5 minutes   **Cooking time**: 5 minutes   **Servings: 2**

Ingredients:
- ✓ 1 teaspoon Seville orange zest
- ✓ 3 oz. raspberries or blueberries.

Directions:
- ❖ Blend the rice in an electric blender until the fluff is dissolved.
- ❖ Add the vanilla and Seville zest. Stir well.
- ❖ Add the walnuts and berries.

Ingredients:
- ✓ ¼ teaspoon vanilla essence
- ✓ 2 cups coconut cream

- ❖ Cover the glove with a plastic wrench.
- ❖ Refrigerate for 3 hours.
- ❖ Garnish as desired. Serve.

Nutrition: Calories 265 Fat: 13g. Carbohydrates: 7.5g. Protein: 5.2g. Fiber: 0.5g.

76)   Coconut pulp Coookies

Preparation time: 5 minutes.   **Cooking time**: 10 hours.   **Servings: 4**

Ingredients:
- ✓ 3 cups coconut pulp
- ✓ 1 Granny Smith apple
- ✓ 1-2 teaspoon cinnamon

Directions:
- ❖ Blend the coconut with the remaining ingredients in a processor food processor.
- ❖ Make many cookies with this mixture.
- ❖ Arrange them on a kitchen table, lined with parchment.

Ingredients:
- ✓ 2-3 tablespoons of raw honey
- ✓ 1/4 cup coco walnut flakes

- ❖ Place the dough in a food grade oven for 6-10 hours at 115 degrees Fahrenheit.
- ❖ Serve.

Nutrition: Calories 240 Fat: 22.5g. Carbohydrates: 17.3g. Protein: 14.9g. Fiber: 0g.

77)   Avocado Pudding

Preparation time: 10 minutes   **Cooking time**: 0 minutes   **Servings: 2**

Ingredients:
- ✓ 2 avocados
- ✓ 3/4-1 cup coconut milk
- ✓ 1/3-1/2 cup of raw cacao powder

Directions:
- ❖ Mix all ingredients together in a blender.

Ingredients:
- ✓ 1 teaspoon 100% pure organic vanilla (optional)
- ✓ 2-4 tablespoons of date sugar

- ❖ Refrigerate for 4 hours in a container.
- ❖ Serve.

Nutrition: Calories 609 Fats: 50.5g. Carbs: 9.9g. Protein: 29.3g. Fiber: 1.5g.

78)   Coconut Raisins cooookies

Preparation time: 10 minutes.   **Cooking time**: 10 minutes.   **Servings: 4**

Ingredients:
- ✓ 1 1/4 cups of coconut flour 1 cup of nut flour
- ✓ 1 teaspoon baking soda
- ✓ 1/2 Celtic teaspoon sea salt
- ✓ 1 button for peanuts cup
- ✓ 1 cup coconut date sugar

Directions:
- ❖ Turn on the oven to 357 degrees F.
- ❖ Mix the flour with the salt and baking soda.
- ❖ Flatten with sugar until started and then stirs in the nut milk and vinavilla.

Ingredients:
- ✓ 2 teaspoons of vanilla
- ✓ ¼ cup coconut milk
- ✓ 3/4 cup organic raisins
- ✓ 3/4 cup coconut chips or flakes

- ❖ Mix well, then place in a powder container. Stir until fine.
- ❖ Add all remaining ingredients.
- ❖ Make small cooookies out this dough.
- ❖ Arrange the cookies on a baking sheet.
- ❖ Bake for 10 minutes until set.

Nutrition: Calories 237 Fat: 19.8g. Carbs: 55.1g. Protein: 17.8g. Fiber: 0.9g.

79)   Cracker Pumpkin Spice

Preparation time: 10 minutes.   **Cooking time**: 1 hour.   **Servings: 6**

Ingredients:
- ✓ 1⁄3 cup coco walnut flour
- ✓ 2 tablespoons pumpkin pie spice
- ✓ ¾ cup sunflower seds
- ✓ ¾ cup flaxseed
- ✓ 1⁄3 cup sesame seeds

Directions:
- ❖ Heat our oven to 300 degrees F. Combine all ingredients in a bowl.
- ❖ Add the salt and oil to the mixture and mix well.
- ❖ Allow the dough to rest for 2 to 3 minutes.

Ingredients:
- ✓ 1 tablespoon gron psyllium husk powder
- ✓ 1 teaspoon sea salt
- ✓ 3 tablespoons coco walnut oil, melted
- ✓ 1⁄3 cups water

- ❖ Roll out the dough on a cookie sheet lined with parchment paper.
- ❖ Bake for 30 minutes.
- ❖ Reduce the amount of food to 30 m weight and let it rest for another 30 m.
- ❖ Crush the bread into small pieces. Serve

Nutrition: Calories 248 Fat: 15.7g. Carbs: 0.4g. Protein: 24.9g. Fiber: 0g.

80)   Spicy Toasted nuts

Preparation time: 10 minutes.   **Cooking time:** 15 minutes.   **Servings: 4**

Ingredients:
- ✓ 8 ounces of pecans or coconuts or walnuts
- ✓ 1 teaspoon of sea salt
- ✓ 1 tablespoon olive oil or coconut oil

Ingredients:
- ✓ 1 teaspoon of ground cumin
- ✓ 1 teaspoon of paprika powder or chili powder

Directions:
- ❖ Add all ingredients to an oven. Brown nuts until golden brown.

- ❖ Serve and enjoy.

Nutrition: Calories 287 Fat: 29.5g. Carbohydrates: 5.9g. Protein: 4.2g. Fiber: 4.3g.

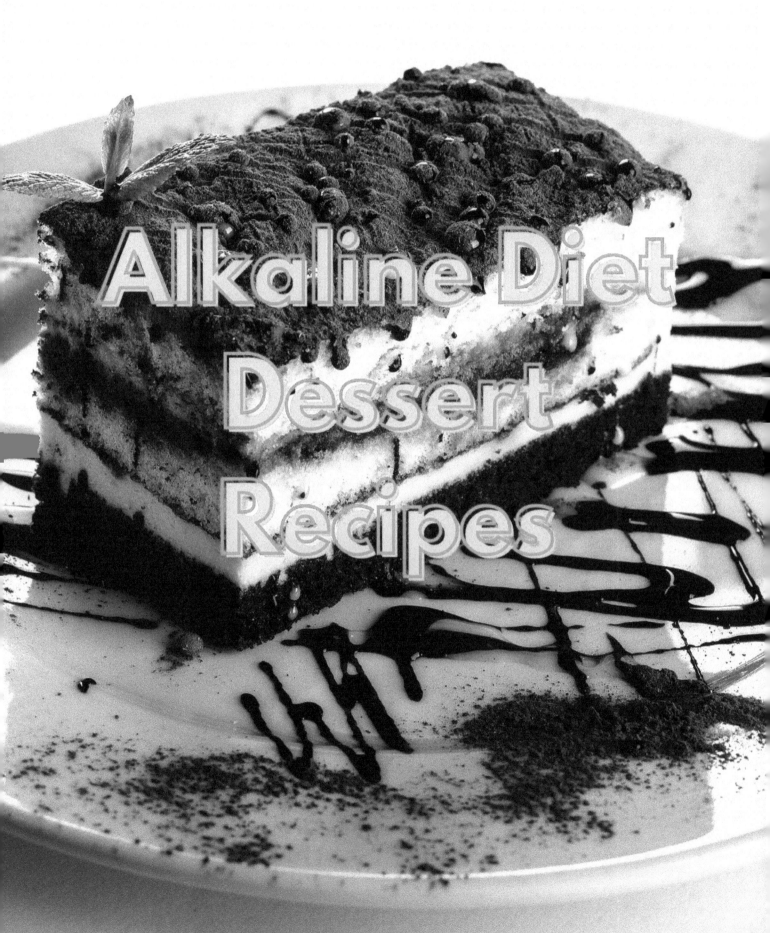

81)   Cracker Healthy

Preparation time: **Cooking time:** 30 minutes   **Servings: 50 Crackers**

Ingredients:
- ✓ 1/2 cup of rye flour
- ✓ 1 cup of flour Spelt
- ✓ 2 teaspoons of Sesame Seed
- ✓ 1 teaspoon of Agave Syrup

Directions:
- ❖ Preheat our oven to 350 degrees Fahrenheit.
- ❖ Add all ingredients to a glass container and mix everything together.
- ❖ Make a ball of dough. If the dough is too thick, add more flour.
- ❖ Prepare a place to spread the dough and cover it with a piece of parchment paper.
- ❖ Degrease the container well with Grape Seed Oil and put the dart in it.
- ❖ RICE the slurry with a rolling pin, adding more flour so it doesn't fall apart.

Ingredients:
- ✓ 1 teaspoon of Pure Sea Salt
- ✓ 2 tablespoons of Grape Seed Oil
- ✓ 3/4 cup of Spring Water

- ❖ When your dough is ready, take a pastry cutter and insert it into the container. If you don't have a pastry cutter, you can use a cookie cutter.
- ❖ Arrange the squares on a kitchen basket and place them in the corner of a ech square using a fork of a skewer.
- ❖ Brush the plate with a little grain oil and sprinkle with a little pure sea salt, if needed.
- ❖ Bake for 12-15 minutes or until crackers are golden brown.
- ❖ Everything that was done was done with the help of another person.
- ❖ Serve and enjoy your Healthy Crackers!

Nutrition: Calories

Helpful Hints: You can add any seasonings from the Doctor Sebi's food list according to your desire. You can make crackers with our tomato sauce, avocado sauce or cheese. Sauce.

82)   Tortillas

Preparation time:.   **Cooking Time:** 20 Minutes   **Servings: 8**

Ingredients:
- ✓ 2 cups of flour Spelt
- ✓ 1 teaspoon of Pure Sea Salt

Directions:
- ❖ In a food processor* blend the spelt flour with the pure salt. Blend for about 15 minutes.
- ❖ Blend, slowly add Grape seed oil until well distributed.
- ❖ Slowly add the soy water, stirring until a color forms.
- ❖ Prepare a piece of wallpaper and pour some parchment paper on it. Dust with a little flour.

Ingredients:
- ✓ 1/2 cup of spring Water

- ❖ Process the nut for about 1 to 2 minutes until it reaches the right consistency.
- ❖ Pour dough into 8-inch pieces.
- ❖ Roll the sandwich into a very thin shape.
- ❖ Prepare a lunch box, cook one tortilla at a time in the microwave for about 30-60 minutes.
- ❖ Serve and enjoy your Tortillas!

Nutrition: Calories

Helpful Hints: If you don't have a refrigerator, you can use a mixer or blender. However, you will have a better result with a food as you have nothing to do with. You can serve the Tortillas with our Sweet Butter Sauce, Avocado Sauce or Cheese. Sauce.

83)   Walnut cheesecake Mango

Preparation time: **Cooking time:** 4 hours and 30 minutes   **Servings: 8**

Ingredients:
- ✓ 2 cups of Brazil Nuts
- ✓ 5 to 6 Dates
- ✓ 1 tablespoon of Sea Moss Gel (check information)
- ✓ 1/4 cup o of agave syrup
- ✓ 1/4 teaspoon salt Pure Sea
- ✓ 2 tablespoons of Lime Juice
- ✓ 1 1/2 cups of Homemade Walnut Milk *

Directions:
- ❖ Place all crust ingredients in a processor and blend for 30 seconds.
- ❖ Prepare a baking sheet with a sheet of parchment and roll out the loose dough with butter.
- ❖ Place the Mango sliced across the crust and freeze for 10 minutes.
- ❖ Place all the glass pieces in a bowl until ready.

Ingredients:
Crust:
- ✓ 1 1/2 cups of quartered Dates 1/4 cup of Agave Syrup
- ✓ 1 1/2 cups of Coconut Flakes
- ✓ 1/4 teaspoon of Pure Sea Salt
- ✓ Toppings:
- ✓ Mango of Sliced
- ✓ Sliced strawberries

- ❖ Place the filling on top of the butter, wrap it with aluminum foil or a food container and let it rest for 3 to 4 hours in the refrigerator.
- ❖ Take out dalla baking form and garnish with toppings.
- ❖ Serve and enjoy our Mango Nut Cheesecake!

Nutrition: Calories

Helpful Hints: If you don't have homemade nut milk, you can use Homemade hemp seed milk.

84)   Blackberry Jam

Preparation time: **Cooking time:** 4 hours and 30 minutes   **Servings: 1 cup**

Ingredients:
- ✓ 3/4 cup of Blackberries
- ✓ 1 tablespoon lime juice Key

Directions:
- ❖ Place blackberries in a medium saucepan and cook over low heat.
- ❖ Stir in blackberries until liquid is gone.
- ❖ Once you've picked the berries, use your blender to chop up the larger pieces. If you don't have a blender, put the mixture in an immersion blender, blend it well, and then return it to the oven.

Nutrition: Calories

Ingredients:
- ✓ 3 tablespoons of Agave Syrup
- ✓ ¼ cup of Sea Moss Gel + extra 2 tablespoons (check information)

- ❖ Add Sea Moss Gel, Key Lime Juice and Agave Syrup to the mixture. Cook over low heat and stir well until dry.
- ❖ Remove from heat and let sit for 10 minutes.
- ❖ Serve with pieces on flat bread.
- ❖ Enjoy your jam!

Helpful Hints: If you don't have Sea Moss Gel, you can omit it. However, the gel gives your skin a thinner, longer-lasting look. Blackberries have a natural pectin, which can have a similar effect. Store this Blackberry Jam in a glass jar with a lid in the refrigerator for 2 to 3 weeks. Do not store in extreme temperatures!

85)   Blackberry Bars

Preparation time: **Cooking time:** 1 hour 20 Minutes   **Servings: 4**

Ingredients:
- ✓ 3 Burro Banas or 4 Baby Banas
- ✓ 1 cup of Spelt Flour
- ✓ 2 cups of Quinoa Flakes
- ✓ 1/4 cup of Agave Syrup

Directions:
- ❖ Set the oven to 350 degrees Fahrenheit.
- ❖ Mash the bananas with a fork in a large bowl.
- ❖ Combine Agave Syrup and Grape Seed Oil to the puree and mix well.
- ❖ Add the Spelt flour and Quinoa flakes. Knead the dough until it becomes sticky to your finger.
- ❖ Prepare a 9x9-inch basket with a parchment lid.
- ❖ Take 2/3 of the dough and spread it with your fingers on the baking sheet parchment pan.

Nutrition: Calories

Ingredients:
- ✓ 1/4 teaspoon of Pure Sea Salt
- ✓ 1/2 cup of Grape Seed Oil
- ✓ 1 cup of prepared Blackberry Jam

- ❖ Spread Blackberry Jam over the dough.
- ❖ Crumble the rice and place it on the plate.
- ❖ Bake for 20 minutes.
- ❖ Remove from oven and let cool for 10-15 minutes.
- ❖ Cut into small pieces.
- ❖ Try and enjoy our Blackberry Bars!

Helpful Hints: You can store this Blackberry Bar in the refrigerator for 5-6 days or in the freezer for up to 3 months.

86)   Squash Pie.

Preparation time: **Cooking time:** 2 hours 30 Minutes   **Servings: 6-8**

Ingredients:
- ✓ 2 Butternut Squashes
- ✓ 1 1/4 cups of spelt flour
- ✓ 1/4 cup of dry sugar
- ✓ 1/4 cup of Agave Syrup
- ✓ 1 teaspoon of Allspice.

Directions:
- ❖ Rinse and peel butternut pumpkins.
- ❖ Cut them in half and use a spoon to de-sed.
- ❖ Cut the meat into one piece and place in a glass container.
- ❖ Cover the squash in Spring Water and boiltare for 20-25 minutes until coooked.
- ❖ Turn off the oven and mash the cooked squash.
- ❖ Add the date sugar, agave syrup, 1/8 pure sea salt, and homemade milk and mix everything together.
- ❖ Crust:
- ❖ Preheat the oven to 350 degrees Fahrenheit.
- ❖ In a bowl, add the spelt flour, 1/2 teaspoon of Pure Sea Salt, Spring Water, and Grape Sed Oil and mix.

Nutrition: Calories

Ingredients:
- ✓ 1 teaspoon of Pure Sea Salt
- ✓ 1/4 cup soy water
- ✓ 1/3 cup of fat seed oil
- ✓ 1/4 cup hemp seed milk Homemade *

- ❖ Reduce the rice into a loaf of bread. Add more water or flour if needed. Let stand for 5 minutes.
- ❖ Spread out Spelt Flour on a piece of parchment paper.
- ❖ Roll out on rolling pin, adding more flour to prevent sticking.
- ❖ Place the dough in a cake pan and bake for 10 minutes.
- ❖ Remove the butter from the oven, add the filling and bake for another 40 minutes.
- ❖ Remove the cake and let it rest for 30 minutes until cool.
- ❖ Serve enjoy your Squash Pie!

Helpful Hints:

87)   Walnut Milk homemade

Preparation time: **Cooking time:** minimum 8 hours   **Servings: 4 cups**

Ingredients:
- ✓   1 cup fresh walnuts
- ✓   1/8 teaspoon of Pure Sea Salt

Directions:
- ❖   Place the new Walnuts in a bag and fill it with three tablespoons of water.
- ❖   Take the Walnuts for an hour and a half.
- ❖   Drain and rinse nuts with warm water.

Nutrition: Calories

Helpful Hints:

Ingredients:
- ✓   3 cups of spring water + extra for soaking

- ❖   Add the soaked walnuts, puree and three times the spring water to a blender.
- ❖   Mix well till smooth.
- ❖   Extend it if you need to.
- ❖   Enjoy your homemade nut milk!

88)   Aquafaba

Preparation time: **Cooking time:** 2 Hours 30 minutes   **Servings: 2-4 cups**

Ingredients:
- ✓   1 bag of Garbanzo beans
- ✓   1 teaspoon of Pure Sea Salt

Directions:
- ❖   Place the chickpeas in a large pot, add the soy water and pure sea salt. Bring to a boil.
- ❖   Remove from heat and allow to soak 30 to 40 minutes.
- ❖   Strain the Garbanzo Beans and add 6 cups of water.
- ❖   Boil for 1 hour and 30 minutes on medium hat.

Nutrition: Calories

Ingredients:
- ✓   6 cups of Spring Water + extra for soaking

- ❖   Filter the Garbanzo beans. This filtered water is Aquafaba.
- ❖   Pour the Aquafaba into a glass jar with a lid and place in the refrigerator.
- ❖   After cooling, the Aquafaba becomes thicker. If it is too thick, boil for 10-20 mnutes.

Helpful hints: Aquafaba is a good alternative for one egg: 2 tablespoons of Aquafaba = 1 egg white; 3 tablespoons of Aquafaba = 1 egg.

89)   Milk Homemade Hempsed

Preparation time:

Cooking time: 2 hours   **Servings:** 2 cups

Ingredients:
- ✓ 2 tablespoons of Hemp Seeds
- ✓ 2 tablespoons of Agave Syrup

Ingredients:
- ✓ 1/8 teaspoon pure salt
- ✓ 2 cups of Spring Water Fruits (optional)*.

Directions:
- ❖ Place all ingredients, except fruit, in blender.
- ❖ Blend them for two minutes.
- ❖ Add fruits and resin for 30-50 minutes.

Nutrition: Calories

Helpful Hints:

- ❖ Store milk in the refrigerator until aged.
- ❖ Enjoy your Homemade Hempsed Milk!

90)   Oil spicy infusion

Preparation time:

Cooking time: 24 Hours   **Servings:** 1 cup

Ingredients:
- ✓ 1 tablespoon of crushed Cayenne Pepper

Ingredients:
- ✓ 3/4 cup of Grape Seed Oil

Directions:
- ❖ Fill a glass with a lid or bottle with grape oil.
- ❖ Add crushed Cayenne Pepper to the jar/bottle.

Nutrition: Calories

Helpful Hints:

- ❖ Close and allow to cool for at least 24 hours.
- ❖ Add it to a dinner party and enjoy our Spicy Infuse oil!

91)   Italian infused oil

Preparation time:

Cooking time: 24 hours   **Servings:** 1 cup

Ingredients:
- ✓ 1 teaspoon of Oregano.
- ✓ 1 teaspoon of Basil

Ingredients:
- ✓ 1 pinch of salt Pure Sea
- ✓ 3/4 cup of Grape seed oil

Directions:
- ❖ Fill a glass jar with a lid or container with grape oil.
- ❖ Mix the seasonings and add them to the rice and lettuce.

Nutrition: Calories

Helpful Hints:

- ❖ Shake and let the oil steep for at least 24 hours.
- ❖ Add it to a dish and enjoy your Infused Oil Italian!

92)   Garlic Infused Oil

Preparation time:

Cooking time: 24 hours   **Servings:** 1 cup

Ingredients:
- ✓ 1/2 teaspoon of Dill
- ✓ 1/2 teaspoon of Ginger Powder
- ✓ 1 tablespoon of Onion Powder.

Ingredients:
- ✓ 1/2 teaspoon of Pure Sea Salt
- ✓ 3/4 cup of fat seed oil

Directions:
- ❖ Fill a glass jar or squeeze bottle with grapeseed oil.
- ❖ Add the seasonings to the jar/bottle.

Nutrition: Calories

Helpful Hints:

- ❖ Close and let oil infuse for at least 24 hours.
- ❖ Add it to a dish and add your "Garlic". Infused Oil!

93)   Papaya Seeds Mango Dressing

Preparation time: **Cooking time:** 10 minutes   **Servings: 1/2 Cup**

Ingredients:
- ✓   1 cup of chopped Mango
- ✓   1 teaspoon of Papaya Seeds Ground
- ✓   1 teaspoon of Basil
- ✓   1 teaspoon of Onion Powder

Ingredients:
- ✓   1 teaspoon of Agave Syrup
- ✓   2 tablespoons of lemon juice
- ✓   1/4 cup of grape oil
- ✓   1/4 teaspoon salt Pure Sea
- ❖   Add it to a dish and enjoy our Papaya Seed Mango Dress5ng!

Directions:
- ❖   Prepare and place all ingredients into the mixture.
- ❖   Blend for one minute until smoth.

Nutrition: Calories

Helpful Hints:

94)   Blueberry Smoothie

Preparation time: 10 minutes   **Cooking time:**   **Servings: 2**

Ingredients:
- ✓   2 cups of frozen blueberries
- ✓   1 small banana

Ingredients:
- ✓   1½ cups unsweetened almond milk
- ✓   ¼ cup ice cubes
- ❖   Pour the smoothie into two glasses and serve immediately.

Directions:
- ❖   Place all ingredients in a high speed blender and pulse until creamy.

Nutrition: Calories

Helpful Hints:

95)   Raspberry and tofu smoothie

Preparation time: 10 minutes   **Cooking time:**   **Servings: 2**

Ingredients:
- ✓   1½ cups of fresh raspberries
- ✓   6 ounces of firm silken tofu, pressed and drained
- ✓   4-5 drops of liquid stevia

Ingredients:
- ✓   1 cup of coconut cream
- ✓   ¼ cup ice, crushed

- ❖   Pour the smoothie into two glasses and serve immediately.

Directions:
- ❖   Place all ingredients in a high speed blender and pulse until creamy.

Nutrition: Calories

Helpful Hints:

96)   Beet and Strawberry Smoothie

Preparation time: 10 minutes   **Cooking time:**   **Servings: 2**

Ingredients:
- ✓   2 cups frozen strawberries, pitted and chopped
- ✓   ⅔ cup roasted and frozen beet, chopped
- ✓   1 teaspoon fresh ginger, peeled and grated

Ingredients:
- ✓   1 teaspoon fresh turmeric, peeled and grated
- ✓   ½ cup of fresh orange juice
- ✓   1 cup unsweetened almond milk
- ❖   Pour the smoothie into two glasses and serve immediately.

Directions:
- ❖   Place all ingredients in a high speed blender and pulse until creamy.

Nutrition: Calories

Helpful Hints:

97)   Kiwi Smoothie

Preparation time: 10 minutes   Cooking time: Servings: 2

Ingredients:
- ✓ 4 kiwis
- ✓ 2 small bananas, peeled
- ✓ 1½ cups unsweetened almond milk

Directions:
- ❖ Place all ingredients in a high speed blender and pulse until creamy.

Nutrition: Calories

Helpful Hints:

Ingredients:
- ✓ 1-2 drops of liquid stevia
- ✓ ¼ cup ice cubes

- ❖ Pour the smoothie into two glasses and serve immediately.

98)   Pineapple and Carrot Smoothie

Preparation time: 10 minutes   Cooking time: Servings: 2

Ingredients:
- ✓ 1 cup frozen pineapple
- ✓ 1 large ripe banana, peeled and sliced
- ✓ ½ tablespoon fresh ginger, peeled and chopped
- ✓ ¼ teaspoon ground turmeric

Directions:
- ❖ Place all ingredients in a high speed blender and pulse until creamy.

Nutrition: Calories

Helpful Hints:

Ingredients:
- ✓ 1 cup unsweetened almond milk
- ✓ ½ cup fresh carrot juice
- ✓ 1 tablespoon fresh lemon juice

- ❖ Pour the smoothie into two glasses and serve immediately.

99)   Oatmeal and orange smoothie

Preparation time: 10 minutes   Cooking time: Servings: 4

Ingredients:
- ✓ ⅔ cup of rolled oats
- ✓ 2 oranges, peeled, seeds removed and cut into sections
- ✓ 2 large bananas, peeled and sliced

Directions:
- ❖ Place all ingredients in a high speed blender and pulse until creamy.

Nutrition: Calories

Helpful Hints:

Ingredients:
- ✓ 2 cups of unsweetened almond milk
- ✓ 1 cup ice cubes, crushed

- ❖ Pour the smoothie into four glasses and serve immediately.

100) Pumpkin Smoothie

Preparation time: 10 minutes   Cooking time: Servings: 2

Ingredients:
- ✓ 1 cup homemade pumpkin puree
- ✓ 1 medium banana, peeled and sliced
- ✓ 1 tablespoon maple syrup
- ✓ 1 teaspoon ground flax seeds

Directions:
- ❖ Place all ingredients in a high speed blender and pulse until creamy.

Nutrition: Calories

Ingredients:
- ✓ ½ teaspoon ground cinnamon
- ✓ ¼ teaspoon ground ginger
- ✓ 1½ cups unsweetened almond milk
- ✓ ¼ cup ice cubes
- ❖ Pour the smoothie into two glasses and serve immediately.

Chapter 7 - Dr. Lewis's Meal Plan Project

Day 1

1)   Blueberry Muffins

23)   Vegetable and berry salad

41)   Mixed stew of spicy vegetables

64)   Mediterranean peppers

86)   Squash Pie.

Day 2

4)   "Chocolate" Pudding.

25)   Grab and Go Wraps

46)   Curried red beans

61)   Quinoa Salad

100)   Pumpkin Smoothie

Day 3

7)   Strawberry and Beet Smoothie

28)   Avocado and salmon soup

51)   Quinoa with vegetables

67)   Alkalized vegetable lasagna

87)   Walnut Milk homemade

Day 4

11)   Orange and Oat Smoothie

31)   Spicy cabbage bowl

55)   Chickpeas with pumpkin

73)   Coconut cookies Chip

99)   Oatmeal and orange smoothie

Day 5

18)   Pecan Pancakes

33)   Vegan Burger

58)   Green beans and mushrooms in casserole

71)   Homemade Protein Bar

82)   Tortillas

Day 6

16)   Hemp seed and carrot muffins

37)   Walnut, date, orange and cabbage salad

59)   Meatloaf of wild rice and lentils

80)   Spicy Toasted nuts

89)   Milk Homemade Hempsed

Day 7

19)   Quinoa Breakfast

40)   Alkalizing millet dish

54)   Spicy baked beans

77)   Avocado Pudding

83)   Walnut cheesecake Mango

Conclusion

I hope this book can lead you to your goals, keeping your desire to keep going high, without making you lose sight of the outcome

This book series is designed to help women, men, athletes and sportsmen, people immersed in work with little free time, etc.

If you recognize yourself in one of these categories or someone you know has decided to take the same path as you,

You'll find the other books in the series in your trusted bookstore, guaranteed!

Big hugs from Dr. Grace!

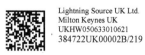
Lightning Source UK Ltd.
Milton Keynes UK
UKHW050633010621
384722UK00002B/219

9 781803 004648